STUDENT SUCCESS
FOR HEALTH PROFESSIONALS
MADE INCREDIBLY EASY

STUDENT SUCCESS FOR HEALTH PROFESSIONALS MADE INCREDIBLY EASY

Nancy Olrech, MSHP, BSN, RN

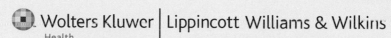

Wolters Kluwer | Lippincott Williams & Wilkins
Health

Philadelphia · Baltimore · New York · London
Buenos Aires · Hong Kong · Sydney · Tokyo

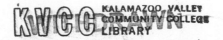

Acquisitions Editor: David Troy
Managing Editor: Renee Thomas
Marketing Manager: Allison Noplock
Production Editor: Gina Aiello
Designer: Joan Wendt
Compositor: Maryland Composition

9 8 7 6 5 4 3 2 1

Library of Congress Cataloging-in-Publication Data

Olrech, Nancy.
  Health professions student success / Nancy Olrech.
      p. ; cm.
  Includes bibliographical references and index.
  ISBN-13: 978-0-7817-8061-2 (alk. paper)
  ISBN-10: 0-7817-8061-6 (alk. paper)
  1. Health occupations students—Life skills guides. 2. Study skills.
3. Success. I. Title.
  [DNLM: 1. Allied Health Personnel—education. 2. Learning—Programmed Instruction. 3. Motivation—Programmed Instruction.
4. Time Management—Programmed Instruction. 5. Vocational Guidance. W 18.2 O52h 2008]
  R737.O47 2008
  610.71′1--dc22

                                                                      2007030886

DISCLAIMER

Care has been taken to confirm the accuracy of the information present and to describe generally accepted practices. However, the authors, editors, and publisher are not responsible for errors or omissions or for any consequences from application of the information in this book and make no warranty, expressed or implied, with respect to the currency, completeness, or accuracy of the contents of the publication. Application of this information in a particular situation remains the professional responsibility of the practitioner; the clinical treatments described and recommended may not be considered absolute and universal recommendations.

The authors, editors, and publisher have exerted every effort to ensure that drug selection and dosage set forth in this text are in accordance with the current recommendations and practice at the time of publication. However, in view of ongoing research, changes in government regulations, and the constant flow of information relating to drug therapy and drug reactions, the reader is urged to check the package insert for each drug for any change in indications and dosage and for added warnings and precautions. This is particularly important when the recommended agent is a new or infrequently employed drug.

Some drugs and medical devices presented in this publication have Food and Drug Administration (FDA) clearance for limited use in restricted research settings. It is the responsibility of the health care provider to ascertain the FDA status of each drug or device planned for use in their clinical practice.

To purchase additional copies of this book, call our customer service department at **(800) 638-3030** or fax orders to **(301) 223-2320**. International customers should call **(301) 223-2300**.

Visit Lippincott Williams & Wilkins on the Internet: http://www.lww.com. Lippincott Williams & Wilkins customer service representatives are available from 8:30 am to 6:00 pm, EST.

PREFACE

To reach their career goals, health professions students will travel through an obstacle course of classes, skills practice labs, and clinical rotations or externships. *Student Success for Health Professionals Made Incredibly Easy* is designed to help students through it with practical study tips that will make them confident and successful students—as well as valuable members of the health professions team—by helping them understand the rules of the game and the skills and strategies they need to win it.

Student Success for Health Professionals Made Incredibly Easy uses the popular "Incredibly Easy" style to make learning enjoyable with a light-hearted, humorous approach to presenting information. Hope, a Health Professions instructor, guides students through the book, offering helpful tips and insights. Along the way, she gets help from three health professions students: Amy, Anthony, and Leslie.

HOW THIS BOOK IS ORGANIZED

Student Success for Health Professionals Made Incredibly Easy is designed to be enjoyable to read, as well as highly informative. The book is divided into three parts:

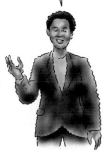

My name is Hope, and I'm your guide to success as a health professions student.

- Part One presents winning strategies for success. Chapter 1 assists students in setting goals and anticipating obstacles. Chapter 2 helps get them off to a good start, and Chapter 3 covers planning ahead, being prepared, and managing time effectively. Part One also contains two Special Sections with extra-helpful information: stress management and grade calculation.
- Part Two helps students sharpen their skills with valuable tips on discovering their learning style (Chapter 4), improving listening, speaking, writing, and critical thinking skills (Chapter 5), developing study skills (Chapter 6), and conquering tests (Chapter 7). This part ends with a Special Section presenting students with strategies for brushing up on their math skills.
- Part Three is important in helping students make the transition from school to the workplace with advice and tips for the

clinical rotation or externship (Chapter 8) and connecting student success skills will workplace success skills (Chapter 9).

SPECIAL FEATURES

Each chapter of *Student Success for Health Professionals Made Incredibly Easy* includes special features designed to engage students with the material and guide them in their study. Each can be identified by its unique icon:

 Winning Strategy–kicks off each chapter with a list of objectives.

 Playing for Real–lets health professions students discuss how they put success tips into practice.

 Tips from the Pros–highlights important tips for student success.

 The Finish Line–wraps up each chapter with a summary of the key points.

Keeping Score–presents review questions and chapter activities.

In addition to these features, *Student Success for Health Professionals Made Incredibly Easy* includes a wealth of fun cartoon illustrations and an appendix containing answers to review and critical thinking questions.

ADDITIONAL RESOURCES

In addition to the text, the following resources are available for students and instructors:

- An **Instructor's Resource Website** with test generator, PowerPoint slides, and Lesson Plans.
- A **Student's Resource Website** with printable note-taking guides for each chapter, printable calendar pages for effective time-management, sample health professions cover letters and résumés, and other student activities.

All resources are available on the following companion website: http://thepoint.lww.com/olrech.

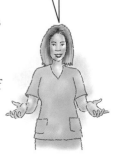

Congratulations on choosing the health professions for your career! I'm Amy.

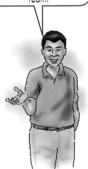

Welcome, I'm Anthony. Glad you're joining the health professions team!

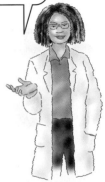

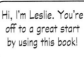

Hi, I'm Leslie. You're off to a great start by using this book!

USER'S GUIDE

Hello, my name is Hope. I am a Health Professions Instructor and I am one of your guides through this textbook. There are a number of features in this **Student Success for Health Professionals Made Incredibly Easy** text to help you learn everything you need to succeed in your studies and in your career as a health professional. Read through this User's Guide to orient yourself to everything the text has to offer. Good luck in your studies!

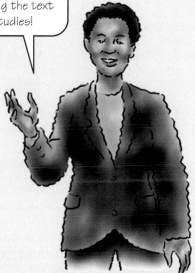

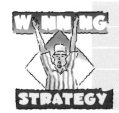

- Know why it's important to be there
- Position yourself to win
- Network to get ahead
- Make a good impression
- Get organized

Winning Strategy Lists set forth the objectives you should meet upon completing the chapter.

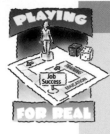

KEEP IT SIMPLE

As a massage therapy student with a part-time job, I find some weeks are more stressful than others. When school gets busy, I try to keep everything else as simple as possible. I do my grocery shopping and run errands before the week starts. After getting home in the evenings, instead of turning on the TV, I sit down, close my eyes, and relax. Even if it's just for a few minutes, it helps me feel less rushed. I also find that I get a lot more done on the nights I don't watch TV!

Playing for Real Scenarios show you how content is applied to real-life situations in the classroom and in clinical practice.

Tips from the Pros offer you expert advice and proven strategies for overcoming study and test-taking problems.

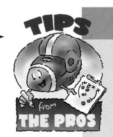

DOWNLOAD THIS! ONLINE DOCUMENTS

Many instructors make their course materials available online. If so, you may need a password to access them. Make sure you get the password on the first day of class. Once you have this password, keep it in a safe place. You never know when you'll need to go to the course Web site to review a course document. Also, if you happen to lose any of this material, you can print out a copy from the Web site.

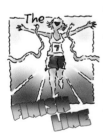

- Use the course documents provided by your instructor to find out what to expect in each course you take.
- Calculate your grades during the semester to make sure you're on target to meet your goals. Don't wait until it's too late for improvement!
- Organize your time by creating yearly, weekly, and daily schedules.
- Avoid procrastination by dividing large projects into several smaller tasks and setting realistic goals.
- Shape your honorable character now, and carry those good traits with you into your health care career.

The Finish Line Summaries highlight the key concepts and skills that you need to master.

Review Questions

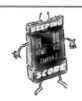

1. How can your syllabus help you be successful in a course?
2. What items do you need to put into your yearly schedule?
3. What challenges have you faced when it comes to honesty, accountability, or responsibility as a student?

Keeping Score Questions challenge you to consider how you will apply the chapter content.

Additional Learning Resources

LiveAdvise Student Success, an online tutoring service, lets you connect with experienced educators who can help you improve your study skills, tackle homework, and prepare for exams. See the LiveAdvise code packaged with the text for more information on this free service.

LiveAdvise
Student Success

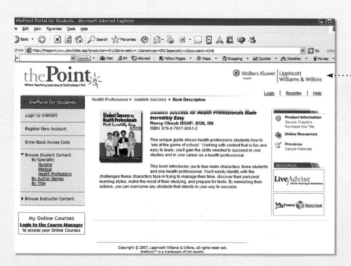

Student Resources are available on a companion website including a student planner, sample cover letters and resumes, links to health career sites, and more! Visit **http://thepoint.lww.com/olrech** for more information.

REVIEWERS

Dana Bernard
President
Boston Reed College
Napa, California

Michelle Buchman
Associate Dean, Education
Everest College
Springfield, Missouri

George Fakhoury
Academic Program Manager, Healthcare
Heald College
San Francisco, California

Laurie Hinze
Dean of Curriculum and Development
Minnesota School of Business
Shakopee, Minnesota

Elizabeth Hoffman
Associate Dean, Health Science
Baker College of Clinton Township
Clinton Township, Michigan

Karen Keden
Corporate Director of Education
GSBC/ACR Incorporated
Visalia, California

Heidi Reihl
Program Coordinator
Rasmussen College
Mankato, Minnesota

CONTENTS

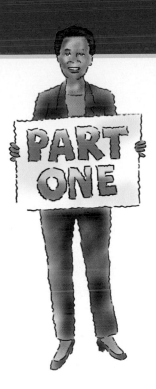

Winning Strategies

Chapter 1

SETTING GOALS FOR SUCCESS

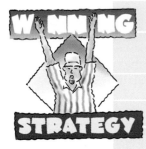

- List your reasons for wanting to continue your education
- Address some of the obstacles that inhibit your success as a student
- Know the importance of goals
- Differentiate between short-term and long-term goals
- Set goals for yourself
- Make a list of things to accomplish during your first week of class
- Know how to become familiar with your campus resources
- Know what to expect from your courses

Way to go! By opening the pages of this book, you've taken a big first step toward your goal of continuing your education. In fact, you've already shown that you're motivated to succeed as a student!

The decision to continue your education may not have been an easy one to make. Maybe you haven't always had positive experiences with school. Or maybe you're worried about whether you'll have the time, energy, or money to stick with it. These concerns are normal—they're also shared by many of your classmates. By using the strategies explained in this chapter, you can gain confidence and sharpen your focus. Zeroing in on what you really want to get out of school will help you stay in the race and cross the finish line.

So in this chapter, you'll take the first steps toward becoming a successful student. You'll think about why you're here—your dreams, the courage you've shown, the choices you've made, and the obstacles you've faced so far. You'll learn about what motivates you and about how to keep a positive attitude. Most importantly, you'll learn how to set and achieve your goals, while following other tips that will help you succeed in school.

Why You're Here

You may have just graduated from high school or perhaps you're returning to school after several years to start a new career. But regardless of your age or experience, why is it important to think about your reasons for going to school? Because these reasons are where you'll find your motivation during those late-night study sessions when you're tired and discouraged. Yes – even the best of students get tired and discouraged sometimes! And those are the times when it is most important to remember why you wanted to do this in the first place.

Taking a few minutes to be totally honest with yourself and really think about why you're here will give you a sense of purpose. Having a purpose that's personal and important to you will help you set goals for yourself. By having real and reachable goals, you'll be more likely to succeed.

> Thinking about why you're here gives you reasons to go after your dreams.

DREAMS

What kinds of dreams led you to this point? Maybe you're interested in finding a career you truly enjoy. Or, maybe you'd simply like to learn more about a subject that appeals to you. There are several reasons why people choose to continue their education. Do you have dreams of:

- improving your lifestyle? You may be the first in your family to attend college. If so, congratulations! The knowledge and skills you'll learn in school will give you more career choices.
- supporting your family? You may come from a single-parent home or you may be a single parent yourself. The ability to provide for your loved ones is an important dream to pursue.

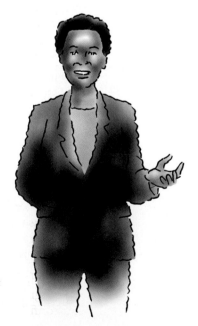

- gaining self-respect? You may wish to continue your education to feel accomplished. Careers in health care provide both dignity and respect.

Whatever your dreams may be, they have brought you this far. Hold onto them, and help yourself reach them by creating a plan for success!

COURAGE

It takes courage to pursue your dreams. You've already shown courage just by being here! Stepping into the unknown is never easy, but you have taken the first step. Right now, school may seem like the unknown. If so, know that you're not alone. Many students feel this way at first.

The best way to overcome a fear of the unknown is to become familiar with it. This book will answer many questions you may have about school. You also will learn simple strategies to help you succeed as a student.

Remember that it takes courage to do something you've never done before. Taking this leap to continue your education will prepare you for other exciting things in your future.

CHOICES

By choosing to continue your schooling, you are making your own path in life. It takes strength to make your own life choices and to work hard for what you want. Just as you've made a decision to continue your education, you can choose to have a positive attitude and be a successful student as well.

Obstacles You Faced Getting Here

It becomes easier to overcome obstacles when you're able to recognize them. You may have overcome obstacles in getting this far. Let's explore this a little bit.

- What kinds of things discouraged you?
- How have people in your life helped or hurt your dream of going to school?
- What life experiences have influenced the way you see yourself?

Recognizing the obstacles you've faced in the past will give you confidence to face future difficulties. You're probably stronger than you think! Although it may not be fun to face challenges, you can benefit from your experiences. If athletes never challenged themselves, there would be no championship games or world record holders. Overcoming obstacles helps you see your true potential.

Ingredients for Success: Attitude and Motivation

Self-image can affect your attitude and motivation. These two things are both very important to your success as a student. If you feel good about yourself and have confidence, it will be easier to develop a positive attitude and the motivation to learn.

Your attitude often determines your performance in school. It's reflected in how much interest you take in your studies or how meaningful your work is to you. If you have a positive attitude about school, you will be able to:

- figure out your responsibilities in the learning process
- set learning goals for yourself
- study for your classes in a more effective way
- improve your grades and performance as a student

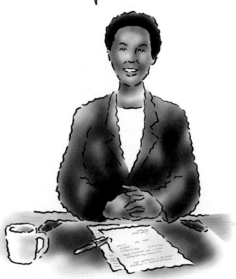

The secrets to becoming a successful student are having a positive attitude and staying motivated.

What type of attitude do you currently have about learning? Find out by looking at some examples of positive and negative traits. (See *Attitude Check*.)

Motivation is equally important. It's what makes you want to accomplish a task. As a student, the right motivation can help you:

- get started on projects and assignments
- move closer to your goals
- keep working on tasks until you succeed

Throughout this book, you'll learn how to motivate yourself to be a successful student.

ATTITUDE CHECK

Is your learning attitude positive or negative?

Positive	Negative
• I'm good at studying. I focus well.	• It's hard for me to study. I get distracted easily.
• I enjoy learning new things no matter what the subject may be.	• I only enjoy learning about subjects that interest me.
• It's easy for me to learn new information.	• It's hard for me to process new information.
• If the instructor doesn't tell me what to study, I'll develop my own studying strategy.	• If the instructor doesn't tell me what to study, I'll be lost.
• I'm confident that I can learn and succeed.	• I'm doubtful about my ability to learn and succeed.
• I have a support system of family, friends, and coworkers—and I rely on them often!	• I don't like to ask people for help, and I don't have a good support system.
• I exercise my mind as well as my body on a regular basis.	• I don't have time to exercise, and I'd rather watch TV than read a book.
• I consider myself an optimist.	• I consider myself a pessimist.

If you have more negative traits than positive, don't be discouraged! Recognizing a negative attitude is the first step toward changing it.

YOUR CHEERING SECTION

As you prepare for the tasks ahead, surround yourself with people who love and support you. A strong support system will help you maintain a winning attitude. And a winning attitude will put you ahead of the game in school!

To become a successful student, seek out support from people and resources, such as:

- friends and family
- coworkers
- other students
- campus discussion groups
- instructors and tutors
- academic advisors
- campus resources (libraries, computer labs, writing centers, etc.)

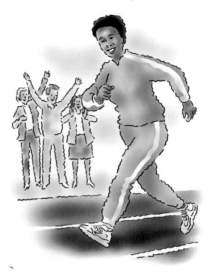

Working hard is easier when you have people to cheer you on!

Keep in mind that you'll need to discuss with your family and friends how things will change while you're in school. Because of your new schedule, you may find that you need extra help with household chores or running errands. If you have young children, be sure to explain your schedule changes to them as well. Let your family and friends know that these demands on your time aren't permanent, and that you're going to need their help while you're in school.

UNCERTAINTY, FEAR, DISCOURAGEMENT—STOP THE CYCLE!

By developing a positive attitude about learning, you can stop the cycle of uncertainty, fear, poor performance, and discouragement. Here's how:

- Take responsibility for your education. Don't simply rely on others to teach you. If a class becomes difficult, ask for help! Your instructor, a tutor, or another classmate may be able to explain difficult concepts.
- Be an active learner. Ask questions about things that interest you. Look for ways to expand your education beyond time spent in the classroom.
- Decide what you want to learn from each course. Then evaluate your courses throughout the semester. This will help you decide whether a particular degree or certificate plan is right for you.

Stress can be another cause of discouragement. When it seems like you have too much work to do and not enough time, stress can be overwhelming. A lot of students experience stress at one point or another. The good news is, there are many different ways of handling stress. Choose a method that works best for you. The way you decide to manage stress will determine how it affects your performance as a student. When managed correctly, small amounts of stress actually help you stay focused and complete tasks. Don't let stress control you. Instead, take control of stress! (See *Taking Control of Stress*, page 27.)

YOU CAN DO IT!

Another way to avoid discouragement is to stay motivated. Use what motivates you to stay focused on succeeding in school. Your motivation may come from within yourself (intrinsic) or from outside benefits you gain from learning (extrinsic). Take the Motivation Quiz to find out what motivates you to learn. (See *Motivation Quiz.*)

MOTIVATION QUIZ

1. I'll spend time studying for my courses because...
   a. I truly enjoy learning new information.
   b. I want to improve my grades and test scores.

2. I've chosen to go back to school because...
   a. I want to excel at something.
   b. it will help me get a better job and a higher salary.

3. Going back to school will demonstrate to others that...
   a. I'm willing to take risks.
   b. I have an impressive resume.

4. Learning new things...
   a. satisfies my curiosity.
   b. gives me a sense of fulfillment.

5. I'm continuing my education because...
   a. I'm very interested in the subjects I'm studying.
   b. I'd like to improve my self-esteem.

If you answered mostly a's, then you're intrinsically motivated. If you answered mostly b's, then you're extrinsically motivated. If you answered a combination of a's and b's, then you're motivated in many different ways!

The Fun Part: Choosing a Motivator

Once you know how you are motivated, you can choose a motivator. A motivator is a reward you promise yourself for completing a task. Choose one and then reward yourself for your hard work.

When trying to decide on which motivators to use for school, think about the tasks you accomplish outside school. Where does your motivation come from? For example, if you volunteer at a homeless shelter once a month, what motivates you? Do you help out because it makes you feel good about yourself? Do you like to talk with the people you meet there? Do you enjoy helping others?

Understanding where your motivation comes from will help you choose effective motivators for school. If you are intrinsically motivated, it may be enough to know that you accomplished a task. If you are extrinsically motivated, you may want to promise yourself a more concrete reward.

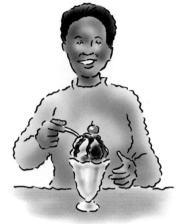

My motivation for working out is the reward of something sweet every once in awhile!

Bonus Benefits

While motivating yourself to do well in school, you'll be accomplishing other things along the way. These long-term rewards may include:

- the ability to apply your study skills to other areas of your life
- a greater understanding of the course material
- confidence and an improved self-image
- improved grades and test scores
- better options in terms of salary and career

Motivating yourself as a student is a win-win situation. Not only will you become successful in school, but you'll be collecting short-term and long-term rewards along the way.

THE BALANCING ACT

You'll need to focus on your studies to do well in school. Worrying about money, your job, or other distractions can hurt your progress as a student. It can be difficult trying to balance all aspects of your life.

If you need to balance going to school with working either full- or part-time, have patience with yourself. You can take courses at a pace that fits with your work schedule. (See *Tips for Scheduling Success.*) Having a manageable daily schedule will help you maintain a good attitude and stay motivated. If you are concerned about working to pay for tuition, there are other options available to you. You may be able to take advantage of financial aid opportunities. Different types of financial aid will be discussed later in the chapter.

Distractions and other responsibilities also can be obstacles to developing a good attitude. Remember: you have to take care of yourself, too! Making sure you are well-rested, eating healthy food, and exercising regularly will help you keep a good attitude. The better care you take of yourself, the better you'll be able to focus on reaching your goals.

Another way to avoid distractions is to set goals for yourself. By focusing on your goals, you will be less likely to become distracted.

Setting Goals

Setting goals for yourself is very important. It does, however, take a little practice. Some people are natural planners and can't help looking far ahead, and if that describes you, you may already feel comfortable setting goals and writing them down. But for those who like to dive right in and start "doing," goal-writing may feel frustrating and dull (at first!). But goal-setting doesn't have to be complicated. Starting small will help you see how easy it is to write goals.

Begin by choosing goals that are simple and practical. By setting goals that are easily accomplished, you will pave the way for tackling larger goals in your future.

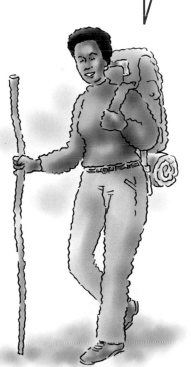

Start with smaller goals and move on to larger ones. If you wanted to become a mountain climber, you wouldn't start with Mt. Everest!

- An example of a good goal for right now might be to become familiar with your school's campus before the end of the first week of classes. This goal is both simple and practical.
- An example of a bad goal would be promising to read your entire textbook before the first day of class. This is an unrealistic goal.

You should give yourself time by starting with smaller, more manageable goals. Once you have accomplished those, your goals can become more complex.

WHY GOALS ARE IMPORTANT

Having goals helps you avoid distractions. Goals keep you from procrastinating, losing your concentration, and losing your motivation in school. In this way, goals are similar to the lanes on a racetrack. They help you stay on track as you run toward the finish line.

Goals come in many shapes and sizes. They can be small or large, easy or hard, immediate or future. Reaching your smaller goals will motivate you to keep reaching for your larger ones. Even completing a small task can give you a feeling of accomplishment. Overall, the more desirable a goal, the more you'll want to reach it.

Goals should have three major characteristics. When setting goals for yourself, make sure they are:

- *Measurable.* All goals need a starting point and an ending point. Be specific. A goal, such as "I want to complete all the assigned reading for my classes this week," is more easily measured than "I want to be a good student."

- *Reachable.* Make sure your goals are realistic. Unrealistic goals can lead to discouragement. Remember, don't start with Mt. Everest!

- *Desirable.* These are *your* goals. Make sure your goals reflect things you want for yourself. Also, make sure your goals are rewarding. Will reaching a particular goal give you a feeling of accomplishment?

LONG-TERM GOALS, SHORT-TERM GOALS, AND EVERYTHING IN BETWEEN

Goals can be divided into four main categories:

- long-term (5 to 10 years away)
- intermediate (3 to 5 years away)
- short-term (6 months to 2 years away)
- immediate (1 day, 1 week, or 1 month away)

Long-Term Goals

Long-term goals are often career or educational goals. These are things you hope to accomplish in the next five to ten years. Consider your long-term goals as your finish line. Any other goals you accomplish along the way should help you make it to the end of the race.

Intermediate Goals

Intermediate goals are the next step below long-term goals. These goals are things you would like to accomplish in the next 3 to 5 years. If one of your long-term goals is to become a practicing medical assistant, your intermediate goals may include completing your education.

Short-Term Goals

Short-term goals will help you reach your intermediate goals. Short-term goals are usually 6 months to 2 years in the future. If your intermediate goals include obtaining a degree or certificate, it may be helpful to have several short-term goals each semester or term.

> At three to five years away, your intermediate goals may seem distant. Don't lose sight of them!

Immediate Goals

Immediate goals are things you plan to accomplish today, this week, or this month. These goals are small tasks that can usually be completed in an hour or less. Your immediate goals should help you reach a short-term goal. For example, suppose one of your short-term goals is to complete a lengthy research paper by the end of the semester. You can start by dividing the work into several smaller tasks that can be completed in an hour or less. These tasks could include choosing a topic, doing the research, making an outline, and writing a paragraph or two at a time. By completing these smaller tasks (your immediate goals), you will accomplish your short-term goal.

GOAL-WRITING EXERCISE

Writing down your goals will help you stay committed and focused on reaching them. Below is a format for writing out your goals. Keep in mind that writing down your goals doesn't make them permanent. You'll be able to evaluate your progress and change your goals if necessary.

In addition, your long-term, intermediate, short-term, and immediate goals should all be linked together. For example, reading 20 pages of course material today (your immediate goal) leads to getting a good grade in the course (short-term goal), which leads to earning your degree or certificate (intermediate goal), which in turn leads to the opportunity to become a practicing licensed professional (long-term goal).

Long-Term Goal (to be accomplished in the next five to 10 years):

1. _____

Intermediate Goals (to be accomplished in the next three to 5 years):

1. _____

2. _____

Short-Term Goals (to be accomplished in the next 6 months to 2 years):

1. _____

2. _____

3. _____

Immediate Goals (to be accomplished today, this week, or this month):

1. _____

2. _____

3. _____

4. _____

5. _____

Is each of your goals:
√ MEASURABLE?
√ REACHABLE?
√ DESIRABLE?

Developing a "To Do" List

Draw from your immediate goals to create a daily "to do" list. The tasks on your list should be specific. They also should have the same characteristics as your larger goals.

- First, they should be measurable. After completing a task, being able to cross it off your list will give you a feeling of accomplishment.

- Second, your tasks need to be reachable, or they need to be things that can be done in an hour or less.

- Third, make sure your daily tasks are desirable. Will accomplishing them bring you closer to achieving a goal?
- One additional characteristic of your daily tasks is they should have rewards.

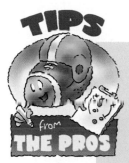

REACHING YOUR SHORT-TERM GOALS

Short-term goals are things you would like to accomplish over the next 6 months to 2 years. Follow these steps to reach a short-term goal:

1. Write down your goal—the more specific you are, the better!
2. Set a reasonable deadline for your goal.
3. Think about possible obstacles to achieving your goal and how to avoid them.
4. Write down a step-by-step process to help you reach your goal.
5. Set reasonable deadlines for completing each step in the process.

IF AT FIRST YOU DON'T SUCCEED, REVISE AND TRY AGAIN

Throughout the learning process, you may need to adjust your goals. Don't be afraid to make changes! Your goals are meant to serve *you*, not the other way around. They are not set in stone.

You may discover better ways of working toward your long-term goals. You may have to find creative ways of working around obstacles. Short-term goals can and should be changed to help you achieve success.

Along the way, you may decide to work toward an entirely different long-term goal. You may even be returning to school without a clear long-term goal in mind. Once you decide to pursue a particular career path, you will need to reevaluate and possibly change your previous goals. If you find something you're passionate about, go for it! Don't be afraid to go back to the drawing board and change direction. Being excited about a long-term goal can be a great motivator.

Reward Yourself!

Rewards will keep you motivated as you work toward your goals. Rewards can be large or small, as long as they are appropriate for the tasks completed. For example, if you do well on an exam for which you've been studying for the past 2 weeks, it may be appropriate to reward yourself with a nice dinner out with friends. A large task deserves a large reward. However, it probably wouldn't be appropriate to reward yourself with dinner out every time you complete a 20-minute assignment! Maybe taking 5 minutes to listen to a favorite song would be more appropriate. In other words, smaller tasks deserve rewards as well, provided that the rewards are smaller.

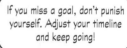

If you miss a goal, don't punish yourself. Adjust your timeline and keep going!

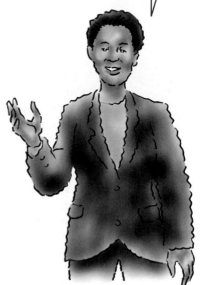

Peer Pressure and Penalties

Another way to stay motivated is to tell a friend about your goals. Having another person to hold you accountable will put more pressure on you to keep working hard. In this respect, peer pressure can be healthy. Just be sure to tell someone who supports your goals. Encouragement from others can be an excellent motivator.

An unproductive form of motivation is punishing yourself for not completing tasks. Punishment often has the opposite effect of motivation. It can discourage you and affect your attitude in a negative way. If you miss a goal by failing to complete a task, try adjusting your timeline instead. (See *If at First You Don't Succeed, Revise and Try Again.*) It's better to accomplish

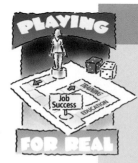

NEW GOALS, NEW FUTURE

When I first started taking courses, my long-term goal was to become an x-ray technician. Then I started working as a part-time administrative assistant in a dental office. I really liked getting to know the patients and seeing them every 6 months. The dental assistants in the office all seemed to enjoy their work. After one semester of school, I decided to change my long-term goal. My intermediate, short-term, and immediate goals all had to be adjusted. But I went back and revised my goals. Now I'm a certified dental assistant, and I love my job!

a goal a bit behind schedule than to become discouraged and give up on the goal altogether.

WILL THIS BE ON THE TEST?

Grades help students measure their progress toward meeting their goals. However, a word to the wise: try to avoid putting too much emphasis on grades. Though that's easier said than done, in long run, learning should be the true goal. Focusing on learning will help you grasp new information and then correctly apply it to situations in the future. After all, you won't be a very effective health professional if you don't learn the material in your courses!

> Obstacles should make you adjust your game plan, not give up on your goals!

Although grades should not be the entire focus of your learning experience, they can, of course, be great motivators. Achieving the grade you wanted on a big test that you studied hard for can help motivate you to study just as hard for the next one. Grades can also help you gauge your progress. You'll feel great when you see yourself doing better and better. On the other hand, if you're not getting the grades you want, you'll know you have to make some adjustments in your approach to your coursework.

To achieve your long-term goals, you may occasionally have to complete some school work that you don't enjoy very much. Maybe it doesn't even seem relevant. But stay positive even when you don't feel like completing these assignments. Although some tasks may seem dreary at times, you will always have motivation if your main goal is to learn. Remember: if learning is itself a goal, you can more easily stay motivated to succeed.

More Tips for Student Success

Once you have your goals written down and firmly in mind, you'll need a game plan for accomplishing them. A game plan is a simple outline of the steps you're going to take in order to win. In terms of your school game plan, one of your first steps should be to get prepared. This means you'll need to accomplish several tasks before or during your first week of class. Some of these tasks are:

- registering for courses
- learning about financial aid
- becoming familiar with campus resources
- speaking with an academic counselor

SPEAKING THE LANGUAGE

Becoming familiar with your school and the resources it offers to students can be like learning a different language. Don't worry! There are people there to help you learn about things like course catalogs and financial aid. If you have questions but don't know who to ask, a good place to start is your school's information office. Look around at the more experienced students who seem like they have all the answers, and remember that each of them had to start at the beginning, just like you! Trust that in no time at all, you'll know your way around and be speaking the language like a pro.

Course Catalogs, Credits, and Confusion

A course catalog describes all of the classes offered in your program. It tells you about the requirements for your degree or certificate plan. And, it also helps you figure out *when* you will complete your education!

Your school may update the course catalog every year or every term. You should be able to get a printed copy or access the catalog online. Be sure to have an up-to-date version handy when planning your class schedule.

Tips for Scheduling Success

If you're attending a career college or technical school, your course scheduling may be done for you. In other schools, though, you may be responsible for registering for courses and organizing your own schedule. The way you organize your class schedule can affect your success as a student. A well-organized schedule ensures that you will be able to devote enough time to each course. There are a few tricks to organizing a schedule that works for you.

- Schedule your classes evenly throughout the week. You can accomplish this by scheduling classes every day. Overloading your schedule to have class every other day can lead to unnecessary stress. Distributing your classes evenly throughout the week will keep you from becoming burned out.

- Make allowances for tough courses. You can do this by scheduling tough courses when you are fresh. For example, schedule challenging classes in the mornings if you are a morning person. Another way to get through difficult courses is to balance your schedule for the term. Try to balance every difficult course with an easier one, if possible, so your schedule doesn't become overwhelming.

- Keep personal commitments in mind when scheduling classes. You may have to schedule your classes around work, family, and other obligations.

- Make informed decisions when choosing your instructors. Certain courses may be offered by several different instructors. When you have a choice, check with other students or your student government association for information on each instructor's teaching style.

Online Courses

Many schools now offer courses you can take online, from the comfort of your own home. Usually, all you need is a computer with an Internet connection to gain access to instructor-led presentations, question-and-answer sessions, assignments, and tests. One obvious advantage of online courses is that you can take courses from home. This virtually eliminates the time you'd normally spend on campus. If you are continuing to work while going to school, taking a course online is especially convenient.

However, online courses have their disadvantages, too. Students who take online courses must have high levels of commitment and self-discipline when it comes to school. Students who have a hard time managing their time and staying organized may find it difficult to keep up with the required reading and complete their work on time. Online courses require that students take more responsibility for their own learning. These types of courses may seem easier, but they can be just as demanding as courses taught in the classroom.

Before deciding to take an online course, think about your strengths and weaknesses when it comes to school. Are you a self-disciplined student? Do you enjoy being able to complete tasks according to your own schedule? Or, do you need the structure of a course that's taught in the classroom? In Chapter 4, you'll learn additional ways of figuring out whether online learning is right for you.

Loans, Grants, and More

Most schools offer financial aid. The federal government also offers several different types of aid. According to the U.S. Department of Education, more than nine million students receive some form of financial aid every year. This may include:

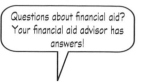

Questions about financial aid? Your financial aid advisor has answers!

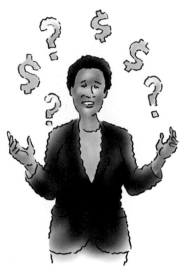

- *Flexible payment plans.* Some schools allow students to make several smaller payments throughout the semester instead of paying one lump sum for tuition expenses.

- *Loans.* A loan is an amount of money given by a lender. Loans must be repaid within a certain period of time, usually with interest. The federal government, as well as private lenders (banks), offer several different types of student loans.

- *Grants and scholarships.* Unlike loans, grants and scholarships do not have to be paid back. The qualifications are often highly specific. There may be a grant or scholarship out there just for you.

- *Work-study programs.* Some schools participate in work-study programs by arranging part-time jobs for students with financial need. Students are paid an hourly rate to earn money for tuition.

For further information on types of financial aid, visit the U.S. Department of Education Web site: www.ed.gov.

Financial aid is available to all students—take advantage of it! Make an appointment with one of your school's financial aid advisors. An advisor can help determine which type of aid will work best for you.

Free Services

Many campuses offer other helpful services to students. The prices of these services are sometimes included in your tuition, or the services are free to students. Some of these services may include:

- tutoring
- learning labs

- writing centers
- computer labs
- libraries
- fitness centers
- career placement services

Need help revising a paper? Visit the writing center! Need access to a computer to do research or work on a report? Visit the computer lab! Although many of these services will be helpful to you during your time as a student, you may find other services useful after you've completed your education. For example, most career colleges offer career placement services and resume-writing help. The people working in these labs and resource centers are often more than willing to help. Take advantage of their advice and expertise.

They're Here to Help

A school's academic counselors are there to advise students. Counselors work with course catalogs and student problems every day. If you have a question about your requirements or if you just need advice, your school's academic counselors are great resources. They can often provide you with information you won't find in the course catalog.

It's also important to establish a relationship with your academic counselors for the future. Some schools offer job placement services as well. Your school's academic counselors may be important contacts to have in your network once you begin looking for a full-time position in your field. (You will learn more about the importance of networking in Chapter 2.)

Special Needs

Some students have special physical, mental, and learning needs. Special needs can include:

- physical disabilities
- mental disabilities
- learning disabilities

Most schools have resources to help meet these additional needs. For example, students with hearing impairments may be able to apply for sign language interpreters to be with them in the classroom. Students who have learning disabilities, such as dyslexia, can work with their academic counselors to find extra teaching and learning aids.

If you feel you need special assistance in school, be sure to set up a meeting with your advisor right away to find out what assistance is available for you. Although students are sometimes required to help pay for some of these resources, other times they are free.

KNOWING YOUR WAY AROUND

If you attend school at a campus with multiple buildings, it's important to know your way around. Not only is it a great confidence-builder to walk into your classes on time and pre- pared, it also helps you avoid stress. You won't have to worry about getting lost or not being able to find the campus library when you need it. Instead, you'll be ahead of the game by knowing where to find your classrooms and where other cam- pus resources are located.

Although you've probably already attended your first class, you will find the tips in this section useful throughout the rest of your school experience. You may even be able to add some great tips of your own.

Don't Get Lost—Get a Map!

The first step toward becoming familiar with your campus is to locate a campus map. Maps may be found in the course catalog, on the school's Web site, or posted at different loca- tions on campus. The school's information office can be helpful in answering questions about student parking and parking permits, if needed.

Be sure to arrive a few min- utes early during the first week of school. It can be difficult getting used to a new routine and remembering where to go. Prevent unnecessary stress by giving your- self extra time to make it to your classes. It's better to be early and calm than harried, late, and out of breath!

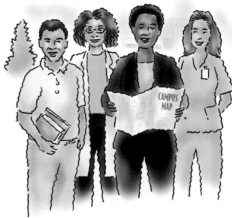

Knowing your way around campus can help you avoid un- necessary stress on the first day of class.

Door #1 or Door #2?

Your course schedule or other information provided by the

school should show the locations of your classrooms. Depending on the size of your school, classes may be held in different buildings, or all in one building. Make sure you know how to read the building and room assignments on your schedule. Part of being prepared is knowing where you're going!

A Funny Thing Happened on the Way to the Library ...

Libraries and learning labs are important campus resources. Most people know what a library is, but what's a learning lab? A learning lab is a place where students can go to meet with tutors or study groups, use campus computers, or use extra learning resources (like anatomical models and skeleton charts). Find out if your school has a learning lab, and if so, find out where it's located before you need it. Remember—your goal is to be prepared. This saves you the stress of hunting for these resources later when you may be pressed for time.

Books, Books, and More Books

Most instructors publish a list of the books you'll need for their classes. They do this because they want students to be prepared. By purchasing your books before the first day of class, you will have a better idea of the material that will be covered in each course.

Some schools offer used textbooks for sale at reduced prices. Because these books usually are sold on a first-come, first-served basis, it pays to purchase your books early.

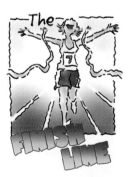

- One of the first steps toward student success is thinking about why you're interested in continuing your education. Your dreams are important in determining your goals.

- Learning to recognize and overcome obstacles will help you become a better student.

- Goals keep you from procrastinating, losing your concentration, and losing your motivation in school. Set goals for yourself so you can stay focused and organized.

- There are different types of goals. Short-term goals are usually set 6 months to 2 years in the future. These goals should help you reach your long-term goals, or career goals. Your long-term goals represent the things you'd like to accomplish in the next 5 to 10 years.

- When setting goals for yourself, make sure each goal is measurable, reachable, and desirable.

- The first week of class presents many challenges. By making a list of important tasks to accomplish during the first week, you can stay ahead of the game.
- You can become familiar with your campus resources by visiting your school's information office. Your academic advisor can also provide information about services your school offers.
- Knowing what to expect from your courses will give you an advantage in school. Seek out information about each course by reading the course catalog and talking to your academic advisor.

Review Questions

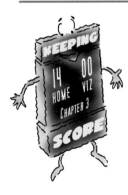

1. What are some common reasons why people choose to continue their education?
2. Short Essay: Write three to five sentences about how people in your life have helped or hurt your dream of going to school.
3. Name several groups of people or resources you could look to for support in your effort to be a successful student.
4. What three characteristics should each of your goals have?
5. Who would be the best person to ask if you had a question about course requirements for your degree or certificate plan?

Chapter Activities

1. First Week Checklist: Review *More Tips for Student Success* and compose a checklist of tasks to complete during your first week of classes.
2. Group Scavenger Hunt: Work as a group to locate the library, campus bookstore, and computer lab.

STRESSED?! WHO'S STRESSED?!?

The word *stress* usually carries a negative connotation. The dictionary defines it as "a physical, chemical, or emotional factor that causes bodily or mental tension and may be a factor in disease causation."

As you have probably experienced, stress can cause physical and emotional tension. It also has been linked to illness. These are all very negative effects. However, there are different types of stress and different reactions to stress. How you choose to manage stress can determine whether you have positive or negative reactions to it.

I Stress, Eustress, Distress, We All Stress!

The two main types of stress are:

- *Eustress.* This type of stress causes positive reactions. Low levels of stress often motivate people to complete tasks, meet deadlines, and solve problems. You may encounter this type of stress every day. Eustress can be helpful. It can stimulate you to accomplish your day-to-day tasks.

- *Distress.* This type of stress causes negative reactions. High levels of stress often cause people to overreact. Distress can cause you to feel nervous and unfocused. It can hurt your ability to participate in and enjoy normal activities.

Symptoms of Stress

Identifying the symptoms of stress can help you manage it more easily. Recognizing stress at an early stage can help you keep short-term symptoms from becoming prolonged symptoms.

Some of these short-term symptoms of stress may seem familiar.

- You begin to take faster, shallow breaths.
- Your heart begins to beat faster.
- The muscles in your shoulders, forehead, and the back of your neck begin to tighten.
- Your hands and feet start to feel cold and clammy.
- You have a feeling of "butterflies" in your stomach.
- You feel physically ill, experiencing diarrhea, vomiting, or frequent urination.
- Your mouth becomes dry.
- Your hands and knees begin to shake or become unsteady.

These short-term symptoms of stress are usually fairly similar for most people. They are also easily recognizable. Short-term symptoms stop occurring once you remove yourself from the stressful situation. For example, you may experience short-term symptoms of stress immediately before giving a speech in class. After your speech, however, your heart rate will return to normal and your palms will no longer feel sweaty.

Prolonged stress can have more damaging effects.

- Your immune system begins to break down as a result of lost white blood cells.
- Free fatty acids are released into your bloodstream, which can clog arteries and eventually lead to a heart attack or stroke.

The symptoms of stress are not always physical. Stress also can affect your mental and emotional well-being. Psychological symptoms of stress include:

- losing your ability to think clearly or remember things
- having difficulty solving problems
- experiencing anxiety or fear
- losing your ability to sleep through the night
- changing your eating habits—either eating significantly less or more than usual

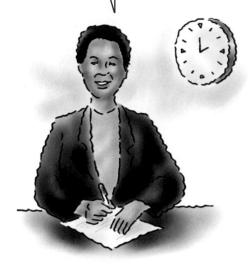

When managed correctly, eustress keeps me alert and focused. It helps me complete projects and meet deadlines.

- worrying
- becoming exhausted

Taking Control of Stress

Just as there are different types of stress, there are different ways of dealing with stress. Several healthy ways of managing stress include:

- setting priorities
- maintaining a healthy body
- maintaining a healthy mind
- depending on others for support

Setting Priorities

Setting priorities helps you manage your time wisely. By determining which activities are most important, you can avoid the stress that comes with trying to do everything. On a given day, your schedule may include attending class, studying, working, spending time with family or friends, and exercising or enjoying other hobbies. Prioritizing your activities allows you to feel satisfied with your accomplishments each day. You may not have time for everything, but you can make time for the most important things.

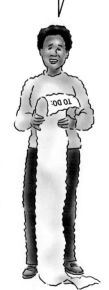

Don't let your daily "To Do" list get out of control. Less important activities can wait.

SIMPLIFY, SIMPLIFY, SIMPLIFY!

One strategy for avoiding stress is to simplify your daily life. The following tips can help you simplify.

- Try to do all your errands in one place. Going to several different locations may help you save money, but getting everything done at the same location saves you valuable time and energy.
- Don't watch TV every day.
- Let your answering machine take messages for you.
- Don't worry about sending greeting cards during the holidays
- Stop attending functions you don't enjoy if they are not required.
- Say *no* to one request or invitation every week.
- Take time out to do nothing.

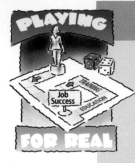

KEEP IT SIMPLE

As a massage therapy student with a part-time job, I find some weeks are more stressful than others. When school gets busy, I try to keep everything else as simple as possible. I do my grocery shopping and run errands before the week starts. After getting home in the evenings, instead of turning on the TV, I sit down, close my eyes, and relax. Even if it's just for a few minutes, it helps me feel less rushed. I also find that I get a lot more done on the nights I don't watch TV!

URGENCY OR EMERGENCY?

Another way to reduce stress is to adjust your schedule to fit your needs. If you have too many responsibilities that you aren't able to manage, try to give yourself more time. You may be surprised to see how many false deadlines you impose on yourself.

For example, if your coursework becomes overwhelming, consider taking fewer courses during the next term. It would be better to graduate several months later than to become overly stressed.

You can also avoid unnecessary stress by being able to tell the difference between an urgency and an emergency. When you feel stressed, divide your tasks into three separate groups:

- *Emergencies.* A task is an emergency if it absolutely has to be done immediately. For example, taking an injured pet to the veterinarian is an emergency.

- *Urgencies.* A task is urgent if it is important, but does not need to be dealt with immediately. For example, taking a pet in for its shots is urgent and should be done as soon as you have time.

- *Non-urgencies.* If a task is neither urgent nor an emergency, it is non-urgent. For example, while it is important to care for your pet, giving your healthy dog a bath is non-urgent.

If you have tasks that don't fit into any of the three groups, remove them from your list. They are not important and should be accomplished only if and when you have extra time. Also, try not to allow other people's urgencies to become your emergencies. When possible, delegate tasks rather than try to accomplish everything on your own.

PROCRASTINATION PITFALLS

Procrastination is another cause of unnecessary stress. If you start feeling overwhelmed by a particular task, stop procrastination before it starts. Large tasks can often be broken down into smaller steps. Completing smaller steps can help you get started on a difficult task without feeling overwhelmed.

Another strategy to help reduce stress is to give yourself some slack. If you often find that you spend too much time trying to complete each task perfectly, you may be guilty of perfectionism. While you may not always have time to complete each task perfectly, you can give it your best effort. Sometimes, your "best effort" means the best you can do in the time you have.

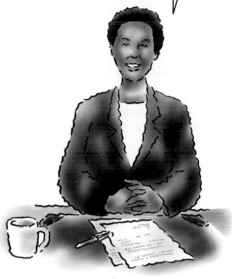

Getting work done on time means having less stress to deal with later.

A Healthy Body Means a Happier You

Stress can take a physical toll on your body. If you take good care of your body, it will be able to handle stress more easily. You will be physically prepared to manage stress when it comes along.

READY, SET, EXERCISE!

Exercising is an important way to keep your energy level up and help you feel good about yourself. Aerobic activities, such as running, swimming, or cycling, strengthen your heart and offer other benefits as well. People who exercise aerobically:

- have more energy
- are less stressed and tense
- sleep better
- lose weight more easily
- improve their self-esteem

Choose an activity you truly enjoy. If you try to force yourself to do something you dislike, you won't be motivated to exercise on a regular basis. Another way to stay motivated is to exercise with a friend or in a group.

For your body to receive the full benefits of exercise, you should work out at least three times a week for 20 to 30 minutes at a time. For even greater improvement, work your way up to exercising four to six times per week. Just remember to give yourself at least 1 day of rest each week.

> Exercise with a friend and motivate each other to keep going!

FOOD = FUEL

Think of food as fuel. Eating breakfast every morning will prepare your body for the busy day ahead. You can give your body the energy it needs by eating healthy foods. This will prepare your body to deal with stress as well.

Vitamin B, vitamin C, and folic acid all help your body handle stress. These nutrients can be found in citrus fruits and leafy green vegetables, among other foods. And the next time you find yourself reaching for something sweet to lift your mood, try eating foods that contain tryptophan instead, such as:

- milk
- eggs
- poultry
- legumes
- nuts
- cereal

Along with avoiding too much sugar, try to reduce your caffeine intake. Caffeine can cause tension and anxiety. Coffee, tea, and certain soft drinks contain caffeine and should be consumed in moderation.

GETTING ENOUGH REST

Rest is also an important key to maintaining a healthy body. When you are well rested, you're able to complete tasks more efficiently. In contrast, feeling tired can increase the amount of stress you feel, which can wear your body down even more. Take cues from your body—when you feel tired, make sure you give yourself enough time to rest.

According to the National Institutes of Health, most adults need 8 hours of sleep each night. But what if you're still unable to get a good night's rest even when you go to bed at a reasonable hour? Other things may be affecting your sleep.

- *Caffeine.* Do you often drink caffeinated beverages in the afternoons or evenings? Depending on how much caffeine you consume on a regular basis, it may be affecting your body's ability to rest at the end of the day. Caffeine is a stimulant that can stay in your system for 6, or even up to 12, hours. Your body may not be able to wind down properly in the evenings if caffeine is still affecting your system.

- *Nicotine.* Nicotine is a stimulant as well. If you're a heavy smoker, you may experience nicotine withdrawal during the night. Waking up multiple times can affect the quality of your sleep.

- *Alcohol.* While having a glass or two of wine with dinner may make you feel drowsy, it can disturb your sleep later on. Alcohol can cause you to wake up during the night. As a result of drinking alcohol before going to sleep, you may wake up the next morning not feeling rested.

- *Food.* Eating foods that cause heartburn can affect your sleep. Not only does heartburn become worse after you lie down, it can interrupt your sleep during the night. Also, the amount of food you eat before falling asleep may affect the quality of your rest. Eating a large meal may make you uncomfortable and unable to sleep well. However, eating too little before bed also can make it hard to get a good night's rest.

On a positive note, a healthy diet and regular exercise are two things that can improve your ability to sleep. Making changes in those two areas may be all that's needed for you to start getting enough rest.

However, if you still have trouble sleeping, you may want to discuss it with your doctor. Getting good rest not only helps you manage stress, it's extremely important to your physical, emotional, and mental health as well.

DON'T FORGET TO BREATHE

If you do experience stress, there are a number of ways to lessen its damaging effects on your body. The next time you feel tense, try following this simple relaxation exercise.

1. Relax the muscles in your neck and shoulders.
2. Slowly lower your head forward.

3. Gently roll your head to the right and pause for 3 seconds.

4. Gently roll your head to the left and pause for 3 seconds.

5. Slowly roll your head down toward the center of your chest and pause for 3 seconds.

6. Switch sides and repeat, moving from left to right this time.

Other popular methods of stress management include:

- therapeutic massage
- yoga
- meditation

Mind Over Matter

Train your mind to focus on the positive. Focus on the goals you want to achieve and imagine how you will be successful. Remember that imagining worst-case scenarios can lead to anxiety and stress. Worrying is rarely productive. But, if you spend your time thinking about success, you will stay motivated to achieve it.

If you are unable to ignore your negative thoughts, try the following meditation exercise:

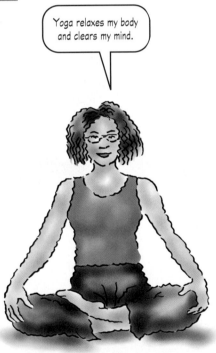

1. Find a quiet place and sit or lie down comfortably with your eyes closed.

2. Begin to inhale slowly and exhale fully.

3. As you exhale, imagine that you are expelling the stress and negative thoughts from your body.

4. As you inhale, imagine that you are replacing the negative thoughts with encouraging, positive thoughts.

5. Slowly inhale and exhale until you feel the tension and stress fading away.

A more conscious method for stopping negative thinking is to say something positive every time you have a negative thought. You may want to repeat an inspiring quote or song every time your mind strays toward the negative. Little by little, you will overcome your anxiety.

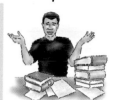

I'm trying to be positive. I'm positive I have too much work to do!

THINK POSITIVELY!

If you want to succeed, you should think like a person who expects success. Some ways to train your mind to think positively are:

- Get excited about upcoming projects and events. Imagine being successful in specific situations.

- Repeat positive mantras: "I *can* do this. I can *do* this."

- Be prepared. Have a "plan B" in case obstacles arise.

- Think of events that cause you to worry as learning experiences. You don't have to do everything perfectly as long as you learn something from your mistakes.

- Think of tests and exams as ways to demonstrate what you've learned. Don't get discouraged for not remembering everything. Completing an exam should make you feel proud and accomplished, not worried and inadequate.

No Man (or Woman) Is an Island

The poet John Donne once wrote, "No man is an island." There will be times when you'll need to depend on others for support. Having a network of supportive friends or family members will help you deal with stress. People in your network of support may include:

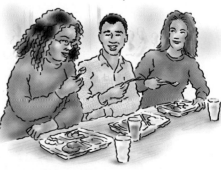

Rely on others for support when you're stressed.

- family members
- friends
- coworkers
- other students and classmates
- members of religious groups
- people who share your interests in sports or hobbies

Discussing your problems or frustrations with others can help alleviate stress. People in your support system may be able to give advice or offer new perspectives. Surrounding yourself with people who care about you will keep you encouraged to reach your goals.

Chapter 2

WINNING TACTICS FOR THE FIRST DAY OF CLASS

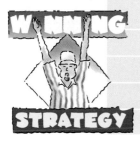

- Know why it's important to be there

- Position yourself to win

- Network to get ahead

- Make a good impression

- Get organized

Contrary to what you may think, becoming a successful student is not all about SAT scores, IQ, or even past grade averages. Much of your success as a student depends on your willingness to take action on winning strategies in the classroom. And there is no time like the present to begin!

In this chapter, you'll learn what to expect from the first day of class. The strategies discussed in this chapter will walk you through the day, from first setting foot in the classroom to taking notes, building a study group, making a good first impression on your instructor, and getting organized. By knowing what to expect and being well prepared, you'll be sure to get the most out of your first day.

Being There

One of the most important steps in your student success game plan is to be there. Attend the very first class, without exception. Of course, you should be there for every class throughout the semester. You have enrolled in your courses for a purpose.

Missing a class here and there will make it harder to achieve your goals. Attending every class should be a top priority. Attendance at that first class period is especially important.

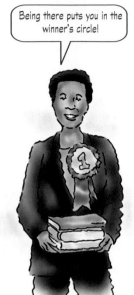

Being there puts you in the winner's circle!

There are several reasons why attendance at that first class period is essential. You will:

- get to know your instructors and other students
- take notes if your instructors lecture on the first day of class
- find out about helpful campus resources
- receive important handouts so you'll know what to expect during the semester

GETTING TO KNOW YOUR INSTRUCTORS

Even if you're a seasoned pro, the first day of class may make you feel a twinge of nervousness. You're starting something new. You're moving into the unknown. You may be wondering what your instructor will be like. Will she be nice? Is she going to be fair? Is she going to present things so you can understand them? Are you going to like and respect her? Is she going to like and respect you? Believe it or not, the instructor is probably nervous, too!

The advantage of being in class on that first day is that you get to see the instructor in action right away. This will help put some of your anxieties to rest immediately. As you listen and observe, you will begin to pick up on the instructor's personality, communication style, and perception of students.

Getting to know your instructor will put you ahead of the game because you'll feel comfortable in the classroom more quickly. In turn, you can begin to concentrate on your studies sooner and more effectively.

TEACHING STYLES

On the first day, some instructors like to share their philosophies about teaching. They'll also let you know how they prefer to run their classes.

- Some instructors like a formal atmosphere where they lecture and students raise their hands during a specified question-and-answer period.
- Others prefer a more informal environment where there's open classroom discussion and students can interrupt at any time to ask questions.

Knowing your instructor's teaching style gives you an advantage in the classroom. You'll learn to anticipate your instructor's next moves. This will help you study for exams, take effective notes, and participate in class. The sooner you can do these things, the easier it will be to do well in the course.

AND THEY'RE OFF!

Another reason you should make every effort to be in class on the first day is because some instructors will start their lectures right away. It's true that some instructors use that first day to introduce students to the course and then let class out a few minutes early. But many other instructors use the entire class time. They'll expect students to start taking notes on the first day. Missing the first class would put you behind in more ways than one.

RESOURCES

On the first day, you'll also find out about many valuable services available to students. There are a lot of resources available on most campuses that you may not hear about otherwise. These resources and services can make a big difference in your student experience.

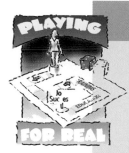

USING CAMPUS RESOURCES

Hi, my name is André. I started taking classes a few months ago to become a physical therapy assistant. Going to school and working at a local restaurant keeps me pretty busy. I even thought about skipping the first day of class because I assumed it would be a waste of time. The instructors usually just talk about unimportant stuff and let everyone out early, right?

I ended up going anyway, and I'm glad I did. My instructor talked about a lot of campus resources I didn't even know existed. He even gave us user names and passwords so we could access a free online tutoring system. It's been great! When I have to work an extra shift and don't have time to meet with my study group, I can log on and talk to a tutor. I never would've known about it if I hadn't gone to that first class. Being there on the first day has saved me a lot of time this semester!

As you learned in the first chapter, many colleges have computer labs that students are free to use. Many campuses also have learning labs and tutors available to help students with their classes. For students with particular needs or disabilities, specially trained staff at the college can arrange for individual accommodations in the classroom. Although you probably know where the library is located, you may need to learn how to use the unique services available there. The first day of class may be your best opportunity to discover how to access some of these very valuable resources.

HANDOUTS

Another important reason you should always attend the first day of class is because that's when the instructor gives out information critical to your success in the course. From this information, you'll be able to chart your moves for the whole semester.

The Instructor's Playbook

Your instructor may hand out a syllabus on the first day. The syllabus tells you almost everything you need to know about the course and what the instructor expects of you. It usually describes the information that will be covered in the course. It includes things such as the grading scale and classroom rules. (The syllabus will be covered in more detail in Chapter 3.)

Other handouts may include schedules of test dates and homework assignments for the semester. You would be robbing yourself of an advantage if you missed receiving this information. Knowing ahead of time what your instructor expects of you will give you an edge when the first assignment is due.

Your Password to Success

Some instructors require that you retrieve their handouts and assignments from a Web site. Be sure to get all the information you need to access the site. This usually includes:

- the URL (Web address)
- your user name
- your password

If your instructor posts handouts online, it's likely that she'll provide the access information on the first day of class. Many instructors spend a great deal of time developing their Web sites to help students get the most from their studies. Chapter 4 will explain further the value of electronic media and instructor Web sites.

Play-by-Play

Most instructors will read through each handout briefly in class on the first day and explain key points. Be prepared to highlight or mark these key points. This is an essential part of your first day, because you will learn about what each instructor considers most important. Some instructors place heavy emphasis on tests and papers, while others place a greater value on participation in class. As your instructor reviews the syllabus, you'll get an idea of what it will take to succeed in the course. Listen carefully to the instructor and be sure to ask questions about anything you don't understand.

A Winning Game Plan

How can you pave the way for success in the classroom? There are several clever tactics all students can use.

- Sit in the front of the room.
- Make sure you can hear your instructor clearly.
- Ask questions.
- Take notes.
- Make sure you can see projection screens and in-class demonstrations.
- Get a copy of each handout.

THE FRONT-RUNNER

Most of us have been to school assemblies or conferences where there are rows of seats. The front of the room is where the speaker's chair or podium has been placed. Everyone coming into the room knows where the front is—and they avoid it! This is very common. As everyone files in to choose their seats, not many people go straight to the front row to sit. Even when there is standing-room-only, seats in the front row often stay empty. We could spend a lot of time analyzing this scenario, but let's cut to the chase: sitting up front in the classroom is actually a very good thing.

Your first step inside your new classroom should be toward the front of the room. Many times, students would rather blend into the background. They don't want to be noticed by the instructor or other students. Although you may have serious

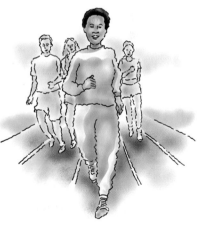

Take a step toward success by being a front-runner. Sit in the front row on the first day of class!

reservations about sitting in the front of the classroom, you'll find that it's in your best interest. Just remember—you're the student with the winning game plan. You're the one who's going to slide into home plate with room to spare.

If you think only the "A" students sit up front, you may be right. But they probably became "A" students by choosing to sit up front, in addition to employing other strategies. It takes effort to achieve success in the classroom. Sitting in the front row is one way to demonstrate that you're willing to make the effort.

TURN UP THE VOLUME

Another clever tactic for your first day is to choose a seat that allows you to hear the instructor well. During the first class period, you'll need to hear your instructor's general overview of the course. This will help you know what to expect over the next few months. If you miss hearing important information on the first day, it can have a negative effect on your overall performance in the course.

The Roar of the Crowd

Classrooms tend to get noisy. One example is when the instructor discusses clinical rotation assignments. This is a very exciting time in health professions classes. Often, before the instructor can finish explaining all the details, students start talking back and forth. Then, they begin asking the instructor questions while other students continue talking among themselves. The noise level rises. Unfortunately, this is when students either completely miss what the instructor is saying or hear it incorrectly. Misinformation then gets passed from student to student.

By sitting near the instructor, however, you'll be more likely to hear her over the noise. Listening carefully involves not only hearing instructions, but listening for answers to other students' questions as well. If you're able to hear clearly, you'll be one of the informed students who leaves class that day knowing exactly when and where you are supposed to go for your clinical assignment.

Listening Skills: Present and Future Use

The importance of listening carefully will be discussed throughout this book. Good listening skills should be cultivated during your time in school. These skills will play a big role in your success not only as a student, but also as a health care professional. When miscommunication occurs in health care, the results can have negative consequences for patients. Not hearing about assignments in school can, at the very least, result in frustration and grades that don't reflect your true ability.

A lot of valuable information will be given out on the first day. The majority of it will be verbal. Beginning on the first day of class, start sharpening your listening skills. Make it a point to listen closely instead of jumping to conclusions. Chapter 5 explains in more detail how to watch and listen for essential clues in the classroom. For now, ask questions if you didn't hear something and write down as much as you can to help you remember what was said. Although information about project due dates and class policies may not appear on a test or quiz, these things are key to your success in the course. Also, by developing good listening habits now, you'll be able to hit the ground running once your instructor begins covering material from the textbook.

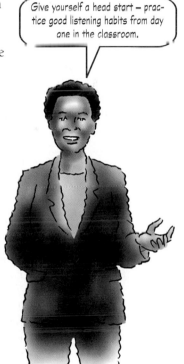

Give yourself a head start – practice good listening habits from day one in the classroom.

ASK QUESTIONS

The first day of class is usually a great time to get clarification from your instructor. After reviewing the syllabus and other handouts, your instructor may encourage students to ask questions. Take advantage of this opportunity! Taking the time now to clear up any confusion about assignments, grading scales, or your instructor's policies will ensure that things go smoothly for you later in the term. Often, instructors won't accept ignorance of class policies as an excuse for late work or missed tests. Know where your instructor stands from the very beginning, and play according to the rules.

TAKE NOTES

Another way to get the most out of your first day of class is to take notes. By taking notes on the first day, you'll ease into a good habit that you can practice during the rest of the course. If your instructor chooses not to lecture on the first day, take notes as a practice run. One of the benefits of note-taking is that it familiarizes you with your instructor's teaching style. Another benefit is that you are more likely to remember information after writing it down. Studies have shown that when students take notes, they remember the information included in their notes 34% of the time. Without taking notes, however, the average student remembers the same information only 5% of the time.

Note-taking often involves listing main ideas and summarizing information in your own words. It keeps your brain engaged and helps you analyze information while your instructor is speaking. There are several other good reasons to take notes during lectures.

- Notes provide you with memory cues to help you review and study the information covered during class.
- Lecture notes let you know what material the instructor considers important. The notes can help you gauge what information will appear on tests and quizzes.
- Taking notes means you'll be more focused during the lecture. You'll be more likely to become familiar with and understand new material.

SEEING IS BELIEVING

It may seem obvious, but being able to see in the classroom is critical to your success in the course. Make sure you have a clear view of the instructor and the front of the room. Pay special attention to where visual aids, such as projector screens, are located. Be sure to choose a seat with an unobstructed view of chalkboards and screens. The instructor may write key terms or main ideas on the board during a lecture. Being able to see this information will be helpful as you take notes.

Charts and Models

Instructors often use anatomical charts and plastic lifelike models, particularly in health science classes. For example, when you are learning about the human skeletal system, a full skeleton model may be used in class. Seeing the model up close will help you learn and remember the names of the bones more easily.

Skills Demonstrations

Skills demonstrations are common in many health professions classrooms. In fact, many health science classrooms are designed specifically for demonstrations and student practice sessions. It's especially important to scope out these types of rooms and choose a seat nearest where the demonstrations are going to be given. This way, you'll be able to see everything being demonstrated.

In class, make sure you have a clear view of the action!

In skills labs, students learn and practice new clinical skills, such as how to take a patient's blood pressure or count a pulse. During labs, you'll be asked to perform the skills your instructor has demonstrated. Having a clear view of in-class demonstrations will make it easier for you to learn new skills and perform them correctly.

TAKE ONE AND PASS IT DOWN

It is very important that you get one of each handout distributed by your instructor on the first day of class. For example, if you have a copy of the syllabus but not the schedule of tests and quizzes, you might be aware of *what* to study, but not *when* to study that material.

If you have time, look over the paperwork before your instructor begins discussing it. Then, follow along as your instructor reviews the information. Even as you're listening, be sure to think of any questions you may wish to ask. Remember, it's better to ask your instructor to clarify things during the first class as opposed to when you find yourself confused later in the term.

Networking

The first day of class is an excellent time to start networking with your fellow students. Networking should be an integral part of your winning strategy—not only while you're in school, but later on in your health professions career. In school, your network will be an informal academic support system that you develop with some of your classmates. This peer network will become an invaluable resource for comparing and sharing class notes. It's also helpful for getting and giving help with your studies and for developing study groups.

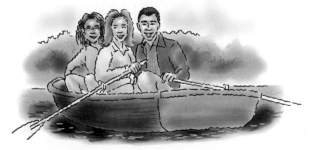

You're in the same boat as many of your classmates. Share what you know and learn from others by networking.

CASTING YOUR NET

Even if you're shy or not very good at meeting new people, you'll find that networking is fairly simple and painless. Begin on the first day of class by introducing yourself to the person sitting across the aisle from you and the person sitting behind you. (Remember—there won't be anyone sitting in front of you because you've chosen to sit up front.) If a conversation ensues, great! If not, you can speak to them again at the next class.

By the end of the first week of class, consider offering a deal to one of the students you've met. Propose that the two of you periodically share or compare lecture notes. Mention that you think it might help both of you understand the material better if you go over your notes together. You also can offer to share your notes if your classmate ever has to miss a lecture. If you're willing to help someone else, that person may be willing to share information with you when you need it.

Because everyone's schedules are already full, it may be difficult to arrange a time to meet. You might suggest meeting in the campus library or student study lounge a few minutes before class once a week. Your new acquaintances might not take you up on your offer right away. If they don't like the idea of networking, they may not realize they're turning down an excellent opportunity. If the first student you talk to is not interested, just move on, meet other classmates, and try again.

BUILDING A STUDY GROUP

Being a part of a study group can help you learn and study course material. Even if your study group is not always able to answer your questions, teaching others can be a good way to learn. Explaining difficult concepts to someone else will help you review the information and get a firm grasp of important points.

If Three's a Crowd...

It's easier to stay on task when everyone in the group is interested in the same thing—studying. If the group becomes too large (more than four or five members), it can be broken down into smaller groups. Meeting with a smaller number of people makes it easier to review all the necessary material and answer each other's questions.

Keeping the Group Focused

When it comes to study groups, remember the four Cs. A successful study group will have members who are:

- committed—interested in learning the material
- contributors—willing to share their knowledge
- compatible—able to overlook differences and focus on studying together
- considerate—willing to arrive at meetings on time

To have productive meetings, your group might choose to designate a "time-keeper." This person keeps everyone moving along at a good pace. That way, your group will be sure to cover the necessary material during each session.

Another way to have successful meetings is to designate a "gate-keeper." This person makes sure the group stays focused on appropriate topics. When people start to discuss things unrelated to the course material, that person can remind everyone to stay focused.

It's your responsibility to prepare before meeting with your study group. You should be familiar with the material you'll be studying together, even if you have questions about it. Your questions may be helpful to the rest of the group. Make sure you can explain other concepts in your own words. Successful study groups have a give and take. If the group answers your questions about one concept, you may be able to return the favor by explaining another idea to the rest of the group.

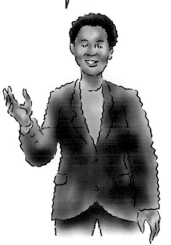

When forming a study group, remember the four Cs. All group members should be Commited Contributors who are Compatible and Considerate.

STAYING SAFE

In the interest of your personal safety and security, remember that it's unwise to meet off campus with people you don't know. In addition, you should give out your personal contact information (phone number, e-mail address, etc.) *only* after you get to know and trust the members of your network.

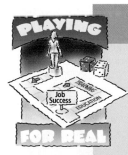

E-MAIL TIPS

Last semester, most of my professors asked students to provide their e-mail addresses on the first day of class. At first, I didn't mind getting messages about assignments and tests by e-mail—it's a fast and easy way to communicate. My problem was that sometimes I would miss e-mails from my instructors because I had so many other messages in my inbox.

This semester, I opened a free online e-mail account that I use for school purposes only. Now that I keep my school e-mail account separate from my personal account, I'm a lot more organized. And I haven't missed any important e-mails from my instructors or from the people in my study group!

Also, your network should not be based on romantic attraction in the classroom. It might seem like fun at first, but you could end up disrupting your own game plan!

Making a Good Impression

Imagine that your first class is drawing to a close. The instructor answers a few last-minute questions and then dismisses everyone. While your first impulse probably involves grabbing your bag and heading for the exit, you have one more task to complete. You need to introduce yourself to the instructor before you leave the classroom. Although it may be intimidating, this is a very important step toward becoming a successful student.

Be reassured—most instructors welcome opportunities to meet their students. They enjoy teaching, and they like to get to know their students. If the instructor learns your name and knows that you're serious about being successful, then you're one step ahead of hundreds of other students. This isn't brown-nosing. It's just good strategy.

YOU DON'T KNOW ME, BUT . . .

"You don't know me, but…" may be the first words that come to mind. That phrase tends to sound self-doubting. Instead, practice an introduction that conveys confidence. Try saying something such as, "Hi, my name is Melody Harris. I'm taking this course as a prerequisite for my Radiology Technician Certification. I'm really looking forward to a great semester. I'll see you at the next class." It's as simple as that.

It's a good idea to plan ahead and practice what you're going to say. If you're especially anxious about this intro-duction, you might want to write down what you'd like to say and memorize it beforehand. When you approach the instructor, relax by taking a slow, deep breath. Then, put on a friendly smile, make eye contact, and make your introduction. If you're comfortable offering a handshake, that would be appropriate, too.

If your instructor didn't cover it in her introduction to the class, now would be an ideal time to ask about the best way to contact her. Should you have any questions over the course of the semester, you'll need to know how to get in touch with your instruc-tor. Some instructors prefer e-mail. Others

Be confident when introducing yourself to your instructor.

prefer a visit during their office hours or a phone call. Be sure to make a note of this information immediately after class.

CLOSE ENCOUNTERS

There are places, such as large lecture halls that hold hundreds of students, where it may not be possible to introduce yourself after class. In these cases, consider seeking out the instructor during his office hours to make your introduction. Your instructor certainly will remember and be impressed with you. And in this more relaxed setting, he may engage you in conversation for a few minutes about your career plans or the class. You may walk away with some interesting insights and valuable information.

CAREER CARRYOVER

Developing your ability to introduce yourself and meet new people is also important for when you begin working in a health care setting. For example, if you plan to work in a clinic as a medical assistant, your job will be to assist the doctor as she sees patients. You will greet each patient, bring him back to the exam room, and ask questions about the reason for his visit. This requires a fair degree of comfort in meeting and talking with people. Beginning to develop this skill now will help you feel more comfortable by the time you have your first real clinical experience. One way to practice is to introduce yourself to your fellow students!

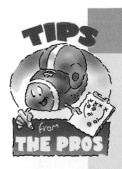

GETTING THE MOST OUT OF YOUR FIRST DAY OF CLASS

Follow this simple checklist to ensure a successful first day of class.

- Arrive early. Allow yourself plenty of time to get to campus and locate your classroom.
- Sit up front. This puts you in the best position to listen and learn.
- Introduce yourself to several classmates. This will be important later when forming study groups or sharing notes.
- Be sure to get a copy of each handout and file papers in an organized notebook.

- Take notes. You will be surprised how little you remember from this first day by the end of the semester.
- Introduce yourself to your instructor. This makes a good impression and lets your instructor know you're serious about the course.

Getting Organized

Let's discuss one final first-day strategy: getting organized. Organization is a key to your success not only as a health professions student, but also as a health care professional. If you avoid getting organized now, you may never have time to do it, and things will descend (or unravel) quickly into chaos.

If you're already a very organized person, you may not need to make any changes in your system for keeping track of things. On the other hand, if you consider yourself less than organized or even hopelessly disorganized, take heart! The following tips and suggestions are simple and easy to implement.

LOCATION, LOCATION, LOCATION

The first step to getting organized is finding or making a place for everything. This means you'll need to find a place to keep the materials and supplies for each class you're taking. To create your organizational system, you'll need the following items:

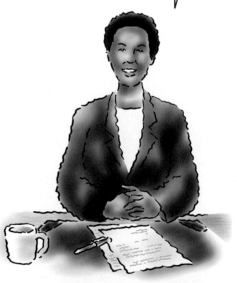

Organization is a key to your success both as a student and as a future health care professional.

- three-ring binders (or twin-pocket folders with notebook fasteners)—one for each class
- sets of tabbed dividers (or colored card stock paper)—one set for each binder
- a pen and/or a fine-tipped colored permanent marker
- a three-hole punch

Dedicate one binder for each class. All handouts, notes, charts—everything related to that one class—will be placed in its corresponding binder. Some students like to use a different color binder for each class so they can tell them apart at a glance. If colorful notebooks are more expensive, don't feel obligated to color-code this way. It's perfectly fine if all your binders are the same color. Just be sure to write the name of the class directly on the outside of the binder where you can see it clearly. Any creative way you can come up with to tell the binders apart is fine.

DIVIDE AND CONQUER

The next step is to decide how you want to organize the material in each binder. You may find it helpful to use the same set of divider names in each binder. This will minimize the time it takes to find things. Use a pen or colored permanent marker to label the tabs on the dividers. Tabbed dividers also can be expensive, but colored card-stock paper is a good substitute. Write the divider name right on the card-stock divider. The following is an example of a typical set of divider names:

- schedule
- syllabus
- handouts
- assignments
- notes

By following this example, your class schedule will be at the front. This allows you to see at a glance what's going to be covered in the next class period. The syllabus needs to be accessible, too, because you'll need to refer to it to find the grading scale and other critical information. Every time you are given a new handout, place it behind the "Handouts" tab. Assignments can be filed behind the "Assignments" tab. The last section is for taking notes in class. Always keep a supply of new notebook paper behind this tab.

ORGANIZING YOUR NOTES

You may prefer to use a spiral notebook, as opposed to loose-leaf paper, for taking notes. Just be sure to keep the notebook matched up to the appropriate binder for each class. The spiral notebook may fit inside the binder for safekeeping. To avoid confusion, use a separate notebook for each class. Mixing notes from several classes will disrupt your organization and derail your game plan.

If you don't have time during the lecture, take a few minutes after class to organize your notes by following these simple steps.

- Record the date of the lecture.
- Number your pages.
- Write down reminders about upcoming assignments and due dates.

THE BACKPACK BLACK HOLE

One final note about organization: beware the backpack black hole. If you are in a rush after class, it may be tempting to gather your papers, shove them into your backpack, and forget about them. The only problem with this method is that when you need to review one of those papers several days or weeks later, you might not be able to find it. A lack of organization makes it easy for important papers to get lost. The backpack black hole occurs when things go in and are never seen again.

This is why you must pledge never to let your backpack or book bag go unattended for more than a few days at a time. Try to spend a few minutes at the end of every day putting stray papers into their proper places. It takes a bit of self-discipline, but your academic life will go more smoothly if you make the extra effort.

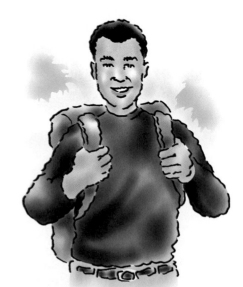

Stay organized to avoid the backpack black hole!

Over the course of a semester or term, those few minutes you spend organizing your paperwork each day will add up to hours of time saved. For example, suppose you need to locate the instructions for a particular assignment. If your handouts are all filed in their appropriate binders, you shouldn't have any trouble finding the page you need. All you'll need to do is open your binder for the class, turn to the "Assignments" tab, and get started right away. However, if your papers are in a disorganized heap in your backpack, you might spend 20 minutes trying to locate the correct handout. In the time it takes to search through piles of paper, you probably could have completed the assignment. Avoid the backpack black hole by taking the time to organize your paperwork *before* it gets out of hand.

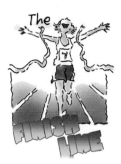

- Always be there for the first day of class. Get all of the handouts and find out about student services and resources. Be ready to take notes!
- Sit in the front of the room. Be one of the first to get all handouts, quizzes, and exams. Have a great seat with the best view and best sound.
- Network to get ahead. Develop good study networks that will help you learn and support your academic goals. Remember to play it safe.
- Make a good first impression. Introduce yourself to your instructor. Show confidence and purpose. Carry this over into your professional life.
- Get organized. Organize your school papers (notes, syllabi, schedule, etc.) for quick and easy access. Avoid the backpack black hole!

Review Questions

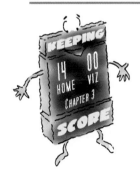

1. What are four reasons why it is important to be in class on the first day?
2. What is one example of a time when health professions classrooms become particularly noisy? Why is it essential to be able to hear your instructor at a time like this?
3. What are four characteristics that members of a successful study group should have? (Hint: Remember the four C's.)
4. How would introducing yourself to your instructor help prepare you for future clinical experience?
5. What are at least two tips for getting organized?

Chapter Activities

1. Getting Organized Checklist: Review *Getting Organized* and compose a checklist of things to do in order to organize your paperwork for each class.
2. Interviewing Exercise: The first step toward networking in the classroom involves introducing yourself and getting to know your classmates. And there's no time like the present to get started! Divide into groups of two and

practice introducing yourself. Then, interview your classmate by asking questions, such as:

- What is your reason for taking this course?
- Have you decided on a particular career in health care (as a medical assistant, laboratory technician, massage therapist, etc.)?
- What do you enjoy doing in your free time? Do you have a favorite hobby?

Finally, introduce each other to the rest of the class.

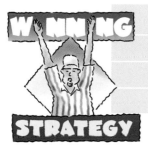

Chapter 3

PRACTICAL PLANNING AND TIME MANAGEMENT

- Know what a typical syllabus contains

- Organize important class dates on a calendar

- Recognize the symptoms of procrastination

- Recognize positive character traits

Being prepared is a large part of learning how to be successful in school. For example, your course documents will let you know ahead of time what each course will cover and exactly which assignments or activities your instructor considers most important. The way you manage your time also will determine your success as a student. In this chapter, you'll learn how to read and use your course documents. You'll also learn how to organize your schedule and use your time efficiently. The section on calculating your grade will help you use your time well, especially if you'll be taking a number of demanding courses. Knowing your to-the-minute grade in each course will tell you where you should focus your efforts.

As you learn how to prepare for and plan your new schedule, you'll also learn about the importance of your academic character. Being truly successful as a student involves more than knowing what to expect and using your time wisely. It also includes learning to be honest, accountable, and responsible. Once learned, these traits will help you achieve even greater success in your health care career.

Planning Pointers

On your first day of class, you'll probably notice a big stack of papers on the instructor's desk. Get ready to collect a good bit of that stack! Although you might start to feel overwhelmed with papers after your first day of classes, every page is important to your success as a student.

WHY ALL THE PAPER?

There's a reason instructors hand out so much paper at the beginning of the semester. They've spent the weeks before the first class planning every class session during the semester. The instructor creates a game plan of the material she's going to teach, the order in which it will be taught, and what you'll need to learn. Then she hands that game plan to you, in the form of course documents. Course documents help you get in the game quickly and easily.

Your course documents may include:

- a syllabus
- a class schedule
- a course materials list
- study guides or lecture outlines
- practice exercises
- assignment instructions

Course documents make life easier for you and your instructor. These documents help ensure that you're both headed in the same direction. This is very important for your game plan.

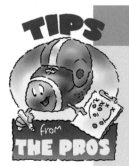

DOWNLOAD THIS! ONLINE DOCUMENTS

Many instructors make their course materials available online. If so, you may need a password to access them. Make sure you get the password on the first day of class. Once you have this password, keep it in a safe place. You never know when you'll need to go to the course Web site to review a course document. Also, if you happen to lose any of this material, you can print out a copy from the Web site.

Course Documents—Game Plan for Your Class

Come to class prepared. You can find out *exactly* what's coming next by reading—and using—your course documents. In fact, reviewing course documents can sometimes help you decide whether or not to stay in a particular class. Look over the books and articles you'll be required to read. Consider how much time you'll have to spend in the lab. See how many exams you'll be taking and how much time you'll be expected to spend on homework. You may find that you've signed up for too many demanding classes during the same term. In that case, you might want to talk to your advisor about your course load and see if you should consider rescheduling one of your courses for another semester.

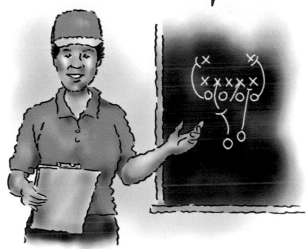

Your instructor gives you a game plan in the form of course documents. Review these handouts so you know what to expect!

Syllabus

You already may be familiar with a syllabus. It's a document that includes the information about your class, just like a coach's playbook. Most instructors hand out a syllabus for their courses. A typical syllabus includes:

- the instructor's name and contact information
- the course name, catalog number, and credit hours
- when and where the class meets
- the goals your instructor has for you (what you will learn)
- the grading policy—how much tests, papers, daily participation, group work, and/or attendance contribute to your final grade
- information about whether the instructor will accept late assignments

Be sure you receive a syllabus and listen when your instructor goes over it. He will clarify anything that seems unclear. If you have questions about your instructor's policies, make sure you ask during or after class. And as with all handouts you receive, file your syllabus in a safe place right away.

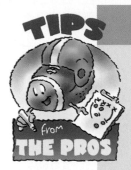

STAYING ORGANIZED

All that paper you get on the first day is important! Look through it all carefully, organize it, and don't lose any of it. It will help if you come to your first class prepared.

As you learned in Chapter 2, filing paperwork in a three-ring binder is a great way to stay organized. It's a great idea to place your syllabus near the front of the binder, because you'll need to refer to it often.

Bring your binder to class so you'll be ready for the avalanche of paperwork. It's a good idea to file all of these important papers as the instructor hands them out. You don't want to misplace any of your course documents or leave them behind in class!

Class Schedule

Usually, a class schedule includes information about:

- what topics will be covered each day in class
- assignment due dates
- test and quiz dates

If the instructor has already organized the class schedule in calendar form, just place it in your binder under your "Schedule" tab for easy reference. If the class schedule is just a list of dates, get out your calendar (which you'll learn to make later in this chapter) and carefully write in the important dates. You might try using different colors, such as red for tests and blue for homework.

Course Materials List

The course materials list includes everything you'll need to participate in each class. This list might include the following materials.

- *Textbooks.* If your school bookstore offers used textbooks for sale, this can save you a lot of money; just make sure you buy the right edition. Some textbooks come with CDs that your instructor may require you to use. Be sure if you buy a used textbook that it has the CD with it.

- *Workbooks*. These may come with your textbook as a set, or you may have to buy the workbook separately.

- *Photocopied readings*. Sometimes, an instructor makes handouts that she gives out in class. Other times, you'll need to retrieve handouts from the course Web site, the campus library, or the resource center. Be sure you have the course materials list with you so you get the correct handouts.

- *Uniforms, stethoscopes, etc*. The course materials list or your instructor will specify where to purchase these items. Ask if there are stores that offer special student discounts.

Sometimes an item on the list is not required—only recommended. Ask your instructor how important it is that you buy recommended items.

Study Guides or Lecture Outlines

Many instructors not only tell you what general topic you'll cover each day of class, but they also provide an outline of each day's lecture for you. This way, you can use this outline as you prepare for class. It allows you to focus your reading and studying on the points listed in the outline. Keep the main ideas in mind as your read, and you'll find you are well prepared for class.

An added benefit is that you will not have to take as many notes during class since the outline is already provided for you! And don't forget to put the study guide or outline in your notebook under the correct tab. You will find it very helpful when studying for tests.

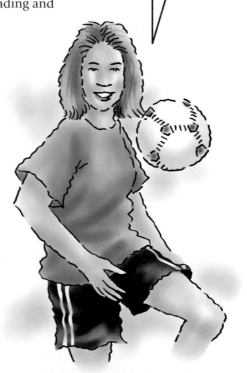

Doing drills and practice exercises is a great way to prepare for upcoming tests!

Practice Exercises

Some instructors provide practice exercises for you. These may be on a handout or on the course Web site. Practice exercises are a great way to drill. If your instructor goes to the trouble of giving you practice exercises for a chapter or section, you should assume that the material is particularly important to know, and that it may be on a test. File these exercises in a safe place so you can use them later as you study. Save any completed exercises so you can check your work when you get graded tests back.

Assignment Instructions

Your instructor may also give you a handout that tells you exactly how she wants certain assignments done. These instructions can include things such as:

- style guides for papers—details on how papers should be typed, how to format your citations and bibliography, what margins to use, etc.
- step-by-step walkthroughs—such as for clinical procedures. Sometimes, many different procedures start with the same basic steps
- research tips—resources for finding information on the Internet or in the library

Remember to file your assignment instructions in your notebook under the correct tab.

HOW DO COURSE DOCUMENTS FIGURE INTO YOUR GAME PLAN?

Successful students have a game plan. They think through what they have to do to do well in their classes. They calculate what it's going to take to get the grade they want. This calculation often involves points or percentages. Unfortunately, many students find grades a source of confusion and frustration. They get their graded tests and assignments back, but aren't sure what the numbers really mean in terms of their overall grade.

This is another time when the course syllabus is very important: it will help you know how to figure out where you stand grade-wise at any time during the semester. But it may take some deciphering! For now, keep in mind that the syllabus has the information you need to figure your to-the-minute grade. In the special section at the end of the chapter, we'll take a closer look.

Due Dates and Deadlines

Due dates and deadlines are two more reasons why course documents are important to your game plan. Turning in work on time helps you stay on schedule and keep up with the rest of the class. Although some instructors have special policies allowing for work to be turned in late, make a habit of turning things in when work is due. If you just can't do it, make sure you turn in assignments within the stated grace period.

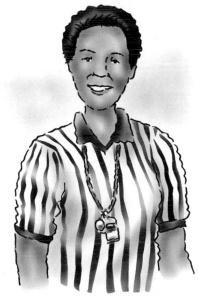

Play by the rules—turn assignments in on time and respect your instructor's policies.

If the instructor doesn't specify whether late work loses points, ask. The answer will be yes most of the time. Why? Late work throws your instructor's schedule off and keeps you working on material A when the class has moved on to material B. The instructor wants everyone on the same page. If you're still working on the last chapter's homework, it means you're not up to speed with the rest of the class.

Some due dates, like the ones for papers and tests, loom large in your mind. You don't need a lot of reminding about them. But there are many other kinds of due dates and deadlines you'll need to mark on your calendar:

- tests and quizzes
- projects and group work
- homework
- field trips and study days
- holidays
- add/drop dates
- last day of class
- registration dates for next semester

You'll learn more about the specifics of planning out your calendar in a later section. (See *Time Management: Flow v. Fumble.*)

Tests and Quizzes

Test and quiz dates should be marked on your calendar. Also, carve out blocks of time beginning several days before each test for studying. If you don't reserve time for studying, it could slip away from you. Prioritize your study time by scheduling it during a time of day when your mind is sharp.

Of course, you also have to prioritize attendance on test days. These are the "big game" days. If there is absolutely no way you can be in class on a test day (due to a family emergency, illness, or other circumstance beyond your control), let your instructor know as soon as possible and ask if the exam can be made up. Many instructors will not allow this, so if yours will, do whatever you can to make it up on the day provided.

Projects and Group Work

When it comes to projects and group work, the scheduling isn't only up to you. As soon as you're assigned to a group, get together with your group members and block out time to work on the project. Start with the project due date and your instructor's recommendations of how much time you'll need to complete the work. Set aside time to work separately and time to get together.

It's tempting to leave this until later—why schedule time weeks in advance? But it's very hard to find one time when three or more people can get together. You and your classmates all have busy schedules. You'll have to prioritize your group work by getting out your calendars and determining a work/study schedule. That way, if someone tries to cancel, you can all remind that person that the date was agreed upon long ago and should be honored.

You'll also have more team spirit if you're working together according to a reasonable plan, rather than trying to cram in meetings with each other at the last minute or to assign work via e-mail.

Homework

Try to estimate how long it will take you to complete a given homework assignment. This will be easier to do as you become more familiar with your instructors and your coursework. But at first, it's probably a good idea to add 30 minutes to your estimate. For example, if you think it should take you an hour to complete a homework assignment, schedule an hour and a half, just in case it takes longer. If you find it really does take you just an hour, you'll have 30 minutes to review, get started on something else, or just take a well-deserved break!

Often, you will have homework based on an assigned reading or lab work. Try to get into the habit of doing the homework soon after the reading or lab work is done, when it's still fresh in your mind. The old phrase, "Don't put off until tomorrow what you can do today," is never truer than in the context of homework.

Field Trips and Study Days

Field trips are invaluable opportunities to visit your future workplace. But they also can wreak havoc on your schedule. Do everything you can to make these trips. Your instructor probably will make clear to you how important it is to be there. Put field trip dates into your calendar so you can prepare for them in advance. You might need to:

- arrange childcare if you have young children
- take the necessary time off work
- ask your spouse or a friend to pitch in and help with any other responsibilities you may have on those days

Also, be aware that you may run late getting back from the field trip, so try to schedule some extra time for delays.

If your school schedules "study days" into each semester or term, make use of these as well. Add these dates to your calendar well in advance. This will help you keep the days free as you schedule your other events and commitments. Try to avoid the urge to use your study days for any purpose other than studying!

Holidays

Holidays are times to relax and have fun. So make sure you do just that. It's tempting to put off coursework when you're busy, thinking, "I'll do that during vacation week." But vacation week often means your family is home, you're traveling, you're working so you can make some extra money, or you're getting together with friends. You won't want to spend that time trying to get work done—or failing to get it done. Block off holiday time and keep it free of any school obligations. You'll need that time to rest so you can come back refreshed and ready to get back to your schoolwork.

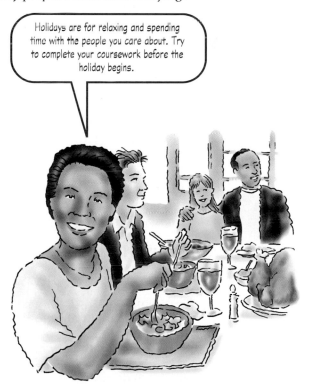

Holidays are for relaxing and spending time with the people you care about. Try to complete your coursework before the holiday begins.

Add/Drop Dates

You can avoid having to add or drop courses after the start of a semester by preparing properly before registration. Before you register for a particular course, gather as much information as you can. (Chapter 1 discussed several ways of doing this.) Then, meet with your academic advisor to determine the appropriateness of each course you plan to take. This way, you can avoid registering for courses you don't need. You'll also want to make sure you won't be taking several very demanding courses at the same time.

But even if you do everything right, you can occasionally run into snags after the semester begins. Maybe after attending your first few math classes, you find that it takes you a lot longer than you thought to complete the homework. It becomes clear that you won't have enough time this semester to devote to the class. For this type of situation, there is a solution—the drop/add period. During specific drop/add dates at the beginning of each semester or term, you can drop or add a course from your schedule without being penalized for it. Mark these dates on your calendar just in case this happens.

Keep in mind, however, that you need to be considerate of your fellow students. Often, there are students on waiting lists who need to take certain courses for their degree or certificate programs. Avoid using the drop/add period as a time to "test drive" courses. You may be taking a spot that someone else desperately needs! Instead, plan ahead before you register and avoid the stressful drop/add shuffle altogether.

Last Day of Class

The last day of class is another important date to mark on your calendar. This date usually occurs several days before the start of exams. While it's important to attend each class period, being there on the last day before exams is particularly important. Often, instructors review material that will appear on the exams and answer questions during this last class.

Registration Dates for Next Semester

The end of one semester or term means it's time to prepare for the next! Mark registration dates on your calendar and give yourself enough time to prepare before registration begins. You might need to research certain courses or set up an appointment with your academic advisor to make sure you're on track for your degree or certificate plan. Remember, if you prepare properly before registration, you can avoid the drop/add hassle after the next semester or term begins!

It's also important to be prepared so you can register as early as possible. Required courses often fill up quickly. If you wait too long, you might not get into a course you need. Stay ahead of the game by going in on the first day of registration and getting it done.

Finally, don't forget about your finances. If you need to save money for the registration fee, you won't be caught unaware if you keep the date in mind.

Time Management: Flow v. Fumble

A full-time student spends about 15 hours a week in the classroom and 2 hours of time preparing for each hour of class work. That's about 45 hours a week either spent in class or preparing for class. On top of these responsibilities, many students also devote time to their jobs, families, and other commitments—that's a full plate.

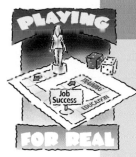

MAKING TIME WORK FOR ME

My name is Angel. I'm 37, and I have two children. I work 30 hours a week at a bank and I go to school every day. My goal is to eventually become a pharmacy technician. In a typical week, I spend 30 hours at the bank, 45 hours doing school-related work, and who knows how many uncounted, unaccounted-for hours making dinner, helping with homework, and doing laundry. I don't have a lot of wiggle room in my life. With so many responsibilities, I'm a typical student. Managing time efficiently is the key to my success.

CALENDARS

People who manage their time well aren't just successful students—they're successful people. They take all areas of their busy lives into account and give each task the right amount of time and attention. The one tool successful people swear by is their personal calendar or schedule.

Creating a personal calendar seems like a negative thing to some people. When they see those days fill up on the page, they feel trapped and overwhelmed. How will they get it all done? A calendar is powerful; it shows you exactly what you're doing each day and how busy you really are. But this is a good thing. Being able to see each week or month at a glance will show you days where you're trying to do too many things at once. A calendar shows you places where your time stretches too thin, and emptier places where you can move some of those tasks.

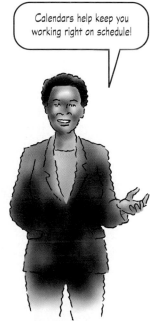

Calendars help keep you working right on schedule!

Most importantly, a calendar helps you to be prepared. If something unexpected comes up, you can consult your calendar and immediately determine how that emergency is going to affect you. A calendar will keep you on track and help you remember important dates. Developing a personal schedule goes a long way toward fulfilling your time management goals.

As a student, you need to do both short-range and long-range planning. You'll need certain items to make this possible.

- a long-term yearly calendar that you keep at home. This can be a paper calendar or an electronic version.
- a small weekly planner that you carry with you, adding new items as you hear about them. When you go home, you can add the new information to your yearly calendar and check for any conflicts.
- a daily to-do list. You'll fill this list with items from your yearly calendar and/or your weekly planner.
- colored pens or pencils for color-coding dates and tasks (if you'll be using a paper calendar)
- a notepad or stack of 3 × 5-inch lined cards for daily to-do lists

You might choose to use an all-in-one organizer. Electronic organizers can store large amounts of information, yet they're small enough to carry with you wherever you go. Just be careful about putting all your information in one place. If you lose it, you won't know your own schedule. It's always a good idea to have a backup, such as a yearly calendar at home that holds all your information.

Managing by the Year

Your long-range yearly calendar should include all your activities, not just schoolwork. The calendar won't do its job for you if you mark next Tuesday's test but not your doctor's appointment scheduled for the same time. Put your whole life—work, school, home—on the yearly calendar. You can use a traditional paper calendar or an online scheduling resource, such as the electronic calendars offered by free e-mail providers.

Use this calendar to record:

- class times
- midterm and final exam dates
- due dates for papers and other projects
- deadlines for completing each phase of lengthy projects
- test dates

- your instructors' office hours
- important extracurricular and recreational events
- deadlines for drop/add
- holidays, school vacations, and social commitments

Off to a Good Start

You'll probably notice right away that the beginning of each school term is a very busy and important time. During the first few weeks of a term, the instructor forms an opinion about what kind of student you are. Are you organized? Do you ask good questions? Do you know what you're supposed to do? Do you complete your work on time? Is your work done correctly? This kind of informal evaluation can help or hurt you. You'll want to be very organized and from the start so you get a good reputation as a student.

Think of the beginning of each semester or term as a fresh start, or a new season. Just as athletes have the chance to prove themselves with the start of each new season, you can prove yourself a good student with each new semester. So start strong!

A Strong Finish

A team that does well in the beginning of the season but loses steam before the championship game is soon forgotten. In school, you need to start *and* finish each semester with the same amount of hard work and dedication. The end of the term is important because you'll be running out of time to catch up if you've fallen behind in your work. Avoid letting your strong start from the beginning of the semester go to waste! Look at your calendar well ahead of time and try to clear less important events from the last few weeks of class so you can focus on a strong finish.

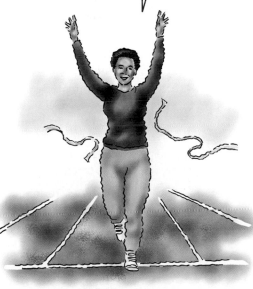

Clear your schedule at the end of each semester so you'll have time to study hard and finish strong!

Timeout!

Whenever you can, try to create free time for yourself. You have to plan breaks in your work if you want to avoid burnout—the fatigue, boredom, and stress that can make life miserable. A break can mean many things: switching from one task to another, getting together with classmates to discuss a group project, or moving from one subject to another.

You can also avoid burnout by keeping your daily schedule flexible. Be realistic when you're planning. If your calendar shows you have 3 days to complete an assignment, avoid cramming it all into 1 day. If you schedule commitments too tightly, you might not complete them on time (or at all), which can leave you feeling discouraged.

Managing by the Week

Keeping a weekly planner helps you tackle the things listed on your long-term calendar, 1 week at a time. At the beginning of each week, you can plan for the tasks that are scheduled for that week. Here are some guidelines to follow as you create your weekly calendar.

- List regularly scheduled events and tasks first (such as class times, mealtimes, and the time you'll spend at work).
- Try to schedule time before each class for a brief review of your notes and to prepare for that day's lecture.
- When possible, allow yourself a few minutes after each class to review and organize your notes. Summarizing is a great (and quick!) way to review the material you just covered.
- Use your time efficiently by grouping similar activities together.
- Make it a habit to complete assignments before they're due. This way, you'll be able to turn in your work on time even if you come across snags in your schedule.
- Plan to study for 50 to 90 minutes at a stretch, and be sure to allow yourself 15-minute breaks between study sessions.
- Base your study time on how many hours of class time you have each week. It's safe to estimate 2 hours of study time for every hour you spend in class.
- If possible, study at the same time every day. Choose a time when you're awake and alert.
- Use "gaps" in your schedule (such as time between classes) as study time. This way, you'll get more work done during the day and you'll have time to relax or do other things in the evenings.
- Schedule at least 1 hour per week to review how you will need to prepare for each class period.
- Be flexible by leaving some time unscheduled.

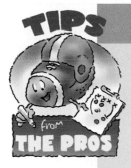

PREGAME PLANNING

It's best to create your weekly calendar on Sunday, before the week begins. Consider it your pregame planning session. Looking at the week ahead will help you spot any conflicts before they occur, so you can reschedule tasks as necessary. And being able to view the coming week at a glance will give you a chance to see how busy each day will be. Try to spread out your activities so each day is just as manageable as the next. You won't want to overload your schedule on Monday only to become burned out by Tuesday!

As you plan out your week, it's also important to be realistic about the amount of time you estimate for each activity. In scheduling time for your commute to and from school, for instance, you should consider things, such as the time of day and amount of traffic. If it takes longer to get to school in the mornings than it does to get home in the evenings, be sure to allow yourself enough time as you create your weekly schedule.

Other activities you should include in your weekly schedule are:

- homework assignments
- papers due
- upcoming quizzes and tests
- assigned readings

Managing by the Day

Once your weekly calendar is in order, you can pull out the next day's activities. You should have a game plan for each day. Every night, get out your weekly calendar and write down the next day's activities on an index card or small sheet of paper. If you use an electronic organizer, such as a personal data assistant (PDA), enter these activities into the next day's to-do list. Include things such as homework, study time, errands, and other tasks that are specific to that day. (See page 68 for a sample to-do list.)

Keep in mind that you can switch certain items around as the day goes on if it will make your day more efficient. The point is to get everything done, regardless of the order in which you wrote the items down. Allowing yourself some flexibility will keep you from becoming stressed.

It's also important to reward yourself for accomplishing everything on your to-do list. Cross off each item after you've completed it. This will give you a visual record of your success. Giving yourself 5 minutes of free time for each large task you finish is another good way to reward yourself—and to make sure you don't overdo it.

Or try this: each day you complete everything on your to-do list, put a certain amount of money into a jar. At the end of the month, use the money to treat yourself. This works better than setting up punishments. Recognize achievement and use days you don't get everything done as opportunities to look at your schedule and to see what changes might make your days more efficient.

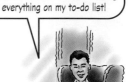

I reward myself with some much-deserved free time after finishing everything on my to-do list!

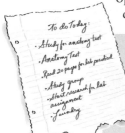

To do Today:
· Study for anatomy test
· Anatomy Test
· Read 20 pages for lab practical
· Study group
· Start research for lab assignment
· Laundry

MAKING A TO-DO LIST

Your daily to-do list should include the personal and academic tasks you need to accomplish that day. The list below shows typical entries on a to-do list. What would your to-do list look like for today?

PRIORITIES

Setting priorities is important to your success as a student. You'll need to set priorities for tasks, class attendance, and homework.

Making Progress

When you have several tasks with the same deadline, it's tempting to switch back and forth from one task to another. This feels like progress on all the tasks—they're all moving ahead. However, you're probably losing valuable time. When you switch from one task to another, you lose momentum. Your brain has to switch gears and begin thinking about a new project. Then, when you return to the first task, you often have to backtrack by finding out where you left off and what other steps need to be completed to finish the task.

In an Hour or Less

If you have an hour or less to work, your priority should be completing a single task as opposed to inching forward on several tasks. Here are a few reasons why it's better to focus on completing one task when you're short on time.

- Completing an activity on your daily to-do list will give you a sense of satisfaction. Once you've crossed an item off your list, you'll have one less task to worry about completing!

- Completing a task moves you closer toward your goals. Think about it this way: Your instructor won't give you credit for simply working on a homework assignment, but she *will* give you credit if you complete the assignment correctly and on time.

Those Marathon Projects

In the case of long-term projects, however, it's sometimes necessary to switch from one task to another. You won't be expected to complete a 10-page research paper in one sitting! If you interrupt work on a long-term project to work on something else, write a few notes on the long-term project before you take a break from it. Your notes could include:

- the goal of the task
- a list of questions you need to answer
- the next step you need to complete

This way, when you come back to the long-term project, you'll be ready to get to work right away. Also, remember to keep all the materials you need for that project in one place so you don't have to spend time looking for them.

Attendance Matters

Class time is important because it gives you a chance to see the material you're studying through the eyes of an expert—your instructor. The instructor goes over key points, provides analysis, and brings ideas to life in real-world applications. In class, you learn what is most important for succeeding in the course and for entering your new career. Attending class needs to be one of your top priorities if your goal is to be a successful student!

Attending class means arriving on time (or even a few minutes early) and staying until your instructor has concluded the lecture and dismissed everyone. The first 5 minutes of class are just as important as the middle of the lecture. During this time, your instruc-

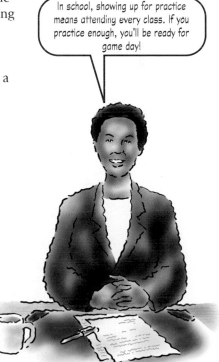

In school, showing up for practice means attending every class. If you practice enough, you'll be ready for game day!

tor might make important announcements. The last 5 minutes of class are equally critical, as your instructor might take this time to summarize important information or answer questions about an assignment. If you have an instructor who is occasionally late, don't use this as an excuse to skip the first few minutes of class. Instead, make use of the extra time by bringing other assignments or notes to review until your instructor arrives.

Show Up for Practice

Really think twice before you miss a class. You joined the team—now you need to show up for practice. Each time you miss class, you fall behind. Even if you keep up with your reading and other assignments, when you skip a lecture or class discussion, you're missing out on an important part of the learning process. Because in class, the information from your assigned reading is analyzed and used as a building block for other, new information you won't get from a book.

Class time offers information you won't get anywhere else. It offers the instructor's own experiences and opinions on what you read in your textbook. During class, the instructor may share journal articles that discuss what you've read and take it further. Even if the instructor sticks to the textbook, you never know where in-class discussion will take that information. You may hear a new idea during discussion that you never would have thought of on your own.

Make it a priority to attend every class. Your instructor will notice if you skip a class or two. Instructors quickly memorize faces, even in large survey courses. They know when you're absent. And even if they don't pick up on your absence at first, if you go to office hours with a lot of basic questions, the instructor will inevitably take out the attendance log to see if you've been missing class. Attendance matters. It's a statement of how seriously you take your education and a measure of your desire to start a new career. If you take your classes seriously, your instructors will take you seriously.

At the End of the Season

Unfortunately, the time most students are tempted to skip classes is at the end of a term, when attendance is extremely important. It's a busy time, and you may decide to skip a class so you can spend extra time studying. But going to class should take priority. Instructors often provide their own review of the course and tell you which items or ideas will be covered on the final exam. If you schedule your study time well and stick with your daily and weekly schedules, you'll have plenty of time to study *and* go to class.

But if you really must miss a class, ask someone in your study group if you can borrow her notes and get copies of any handouts for that day. See if that student can spend 5 minutes with you describing the discussion that took place. That way, you'll get at least some of the information you missed.

Doing Homework

Homework usually includes writing or reading assignments. Written assignments show your instructor how well you understand the material. They show how much work you've finished and whether you know exactly what you're doing.

Reading assignments don't give the instructor immediate feedback on your performance, but most instructors consider them to be just as important as written work. You might see questions about reading assignments on later quizzes or tests. Also, your instructor may base class discussions on the assigned readings. During discussions, the instructor can use student responses to determine how well the class has learned the material. If your instructor relies on class discussions, be sure to complete the reading so you'll be prepared to participate!

No Pain, No Gain

To gain benefits from doing your homework assignments, you first have to know what they are and when they're due. As you learned earlier in this chapter, assignment due dates are often provided in the form of a class schedule or similar handout. Because you were organized enough to place these handouts in your binder when you received them, locating the information you need should be easy. Just remember to make a note of assignments in your weekly planner and transfer these tasks to your daily to-do list so you can complete them on time.

Other Responsibilities

Like most students, you probably have family, work, or other responsibilities outside of school. Sometimes, you might have to put off doing homework because of a more pressing obligation. This is understandable, and when this happens, it's okay to adjust your schedule. The key is to stay balanced. When you postpone working on a homework assignment because of another responsibility, be sure to make time in your schedule to complete the assignment before it's due.

Try to keep yourself from overdoing it at work or at home if you find that your schoolwork is suffering. As you learned in Chapter 1, it's important to have a strong support system of family, friends, coworkers—and even your employer—while you're in school. When you surround yourself with people who are willing to pitch in and help you reach your goals, it won't be so tempting to let yourself fall behind in your studies!

PROCRASTINATION

Procrastination is so common that we tend to fall into its trap easily, thinking it's not so bad to put things off. But procrastination is just a fancy word for wasting time. And you know that wasting time harms your success as a student. It leads to missed opportunities, poor performance, low self-esteem, and heavy stress.

When you procrastinate, you spend your time worrying instead of working. The task you postponed starts to weigh heavily on your mind. You imagine how hard it will be, and you start to dread it. But this doesn't have to be the case! There are several steps you can take to recognize procrastination and put a stop to it.

Prioritize, Prioritize, Prioritize

One habit that leads to procrastination is failing to prioritize your tasks correctly. Putting low-priority (non-urgent) tasks ahead of high-priority (urgent) tasks is all too common. There are many familiar excuses for avoiding important work, such as:

- I'm not in the mood. I have to wait until I'm in the mood, or I won't do well.
- I feel like taking a break to celebrate finishing one chapter. I'll read the second chapter after that.
- I'll do it tomorrow.
- I've got plenty of time—there's no rush.
- I don't know where to start.
- I like working under pressure.
- I need to do other things first, or I won't be able to concentrate.

What's the thinking behind all these excuses? Usually, it's a lack of confidence. You might think the task is going to be too hard. You worry about being able to do it right. You fear it will take forever. You read every bit of material you can to "prepare" for the project—buying time before you have to begin. When you're worried about the outcome of a project, it's hard to find the motivation to get started.

Now's the time to shake the lack of confidence that wastes your valuable time. First, remember who you are—a motivated, efficient student dedicated to your education and your future career. Then, remember why you're doing the project—to get the information and experience you'll need in your new career. Last, remember that nothing is as hard as it seems. You just have to start. The sooner you start, the sooner you'll be done!

Here are some ways to get started on that big project right away.

- Do a little bit at a time.
- Juggle your deadlines.
- Set realistic goals.
- Stay focused.
- Be confident about your decisions.
- Keep your goals in mind.

A Little at a Time

Try spending just 5 minutes on the project you've been dreading and putting off. Once you start, you'll probably find that you can keep working beyond 5 minutes.

Juggling Deadlines

Occasionally, the problem is having several deadlines in the same week. It's tempting to do the easier projects first, "leaving time" for the hardest one at the end of the week. But it would be wise to clear the most difficult project out of the way first. With the pressure off, you'll be able to relax a bit and work on the smaller projects.

If the projects are equally large, try parceling out the work. Set apart small tasks that can be done quickly for each project. Once you have those small tasks out of the way, you can focus all your energy on one project first, then the other. Completing several small tasks gives you confidence and gets you closer to being done.

Keep It Real

What if the problem is unrealistic goals? Some students don't start projects in time because they set standards that are too high (by accepting nothing less than 100% or

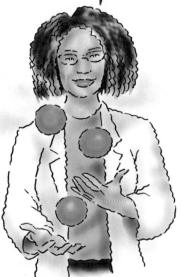

When juggling deadlines, divide your work into smaller tasks to make it more manageable.

vowing to do something better and faster than everyone else in the class). They're afraid they won't live up to those high standards. Or they won't stop working until they feel the project is perfect, which causes them to miss the deadline.

What is the solution? Weigh the consequences of handing in what you think is an imperfect project against the consequences of handing it in late or not at all. A passing grade for an imperfect assignment is better than a zero for not handing it in at all.

Stay Focused

Where there's distraction, there's procrastination. Your mind will seek out distractions to avoid starting a project. You have to fight it. Get your game face on! Work on the project in a quiet area that is free from distractions. If you're in the kitchen, you might eat or do dishes as opposed to working. If you're in the living room, you might be distracted by the TV. (Chapter 6 provides additional tips for choosing a good study space and staying focused.)

Another good way to avoid distractions is to make sure you have all the materials you need before sitting down to begin a project. It can be disruptive to your train of thought if you're constantly getting up to find another resource. Even small interruptions can cause you to lose momentum. Instead, gather your materials before you get started and then prepare to focus!

Be Confident About Your Decisions

Uncertainty leads to indecisiveness, which usually ends in procrastination. For example, if you're not sure which topic to choose for a project, it becomes easier to put off starting the project. When this happens, remind yourself that you have to be decisive to become a successful student. Have confidence in yourself! The next time you're feeling lost and having a hard time choosing a topic, use these tips to help you get started.

- Brainstorm for ideas with other students.
- Ask your instructor for suggestions.
- Research several topics that might interest you.

Keep Your Eyes on the Prize

Remember the long-term and short-term goals you wrote down in Chapter 1? By keeping these goals in mind, you'll have an easier time staying on track and avoiding procrastination. When you're thinking about your goals, an assignment becomes more than just another task that has to be gotten through. It becomes your ticket to reaching your short-term goal of passing the course. And passing the course moves you closer toward your long-term goal of eventually becoming a licensed professional.

By defining your goals, you can give yourself the motivation you need to complete assignments that you might otherwise put off. Review your goals whenever you feel the urge to procrastinate. Also, looking at your goals is a good way to get back on track if you notice that you're putting too much energy into one assignment at the expense of other projects and commitments. Your goals will help you stay balanced and moving forward to greater success.

Academic Character

The character you have as a student is the character you'll have as a health care professional. You're facing the challenges of your new career today—learning new information, dealing with associates (the classmates of today are the coworkers of tomorrow), and taking responsibility for your work and your decisions.

Working in health care is different than working in any other profession. You are entrusted with personal information on a daily basis. One day, you might listen to very private concerns, examine people's bodies, or handle their financial information. You must take these responsibilities seriously. People share information in a health care setting that they would never share anywhere else. You may learn things about patients that their own families don't know. The trust your patients put in you is critically important and sacred.

In school, you should develop the characteristics you'll need to become a trusted health care professional. There are three main characteristics to develop.

- *Honesty*. Be someone your instructors, patients, and colleagues can trust.

- *Accountability*. Be able to account for what you do at school and work all day, every day.

- *Responsibility*. Be someone who never tries to get out of doing work.

HONESTY

You should be familiar with academic honesty. It boils down to doing your own work: no plagiarism

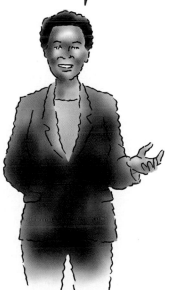

Your personal character matters when it comes to being a health care professional.

from books or articles, no copying a classmate's work, and no cheating on tests or assignments.

But honesty takes on new meaning in a health care setting. How would you feel if your doctor or nurse had passed a final by cheating? Or plagiarized his final paper? Or had a lab partner who did all the work for him? You would think that particular doctor or nurse was not qualified to answer your health questions or treat you. You would be right. Doing your own work is never more important than when you're learning to care for someone's health. You have to know the material—you won't be able to fake it in a professional setting.

Make a concrete commitment to honesty.

- Do your own work.

- Avoid plagiarizing. Make sure you understand ideas well enough to put them in your own words.

- Own up to work you haven't done. If you're not prepared for a class or lab, admit it. Promise to make it up and that you won't let it happen again—and don't let it happen again!

You may be honest, and you may find that some of your classmates are not. Make a stand here, too.

- Expect the members of your study group to do their own work.

- Don't let anyone copy your work. Sharing notes is not the same as letting someone copy an assignment you completed. Notes are raw material, not finished work that uses ideas and analysis.

- Don't let classmates force you to cover for them if they haven't done their work. You don't have to be confrontational, just firm.

One of the biggest mistakes people working in a health care facility can make is gossiping about patient information. For example, suppose a coworker asks you a casual question about a patient. Even thought it may seem like a harmless question, keep your lips sealed. Not only does sharing private patient information violate the patient's privacy, it can get you fired. You never know who is listening or where else that information might travel. Only share confidential information that is required for providing care of the patient.

Whenever you're in doubt about whether something you're doing is honest, think about it this way: would you want your doctor or nurse to do what you're thinking of doing? If the answer is no, don't do it. Period.

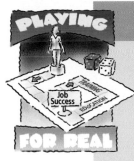

NO CHEATING

I work at a local hospital on Tuesdays and Thursdays, and the staff there know I'm a health care student. One day, a nurse's assistant was telling me about a patient of his. He likes to quiz me, so he gave me the patient's chart and asked me what I thought. It was tempting to show off what I've learned. But I gave the chart right back without looking at it. I reminded him of HIPAA and told him I couldn't look at a patient's private information (see more about HIPAA in Chapter 8).

ACCOUNTABILITY

Being accountable means you have to be able to explain your actions. You are held to certain standards. An employee, for instance, is accountable to her supervisor. As a student, you are accountable to:

- your instructor
- your classmates
- yourself

You have to be able to explain to your instructor the quality of your work, your attendance, and your attitude. This means things like owning up to whether or not you studied and explaining why you turned in an assignment late.

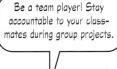

Be a team player! Stay accountable to your class-mates during group projects.

How do classmates come into play? If you're working on a group project, you need to be able to tell the other group members about the work you've done toward the group goal—or why you didn't do that work. You also need to be able to help everyone learn by participating in group discussions.

You're accountable to yourself in that you're working toward your

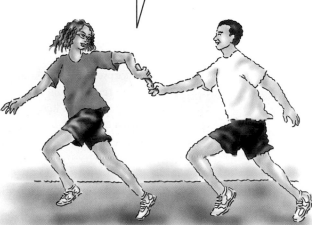

own goals. If you're letting yourself down, you have to be able to admit it and then ask yourself why.

As a health care professional, you'll be accountable to:

- the patient
- your supervisor
- your workplace

Helping patients is the reason why everyone at a clinic, doctor's office, or hospital is there. You are accountable to your patients.

When it comes to your supervisor, you'll have to answer questions about the work you've done. For example, a medical assistant might have to answer questions such as:

- Did you file all the paperwork?
- Did you check every vital sign?
- Did you label all specimens?
- Did you write down symptoms correctly and pass them on to the nurse or doctor?

And, more importantly, did you do all this correctly and on time?

Finally, you are accountable to your workplace—the health care facility where you work. Always work and act as though you might be called upon to explain your actions.

The way to make accountability easy is to toe the line. Do what you're supposed to do when you're supposed to do it. Be focused on your work when you're at work. If you form that habit now while in school, all the tips you learn about prioritizing and scheduling will come to your rescue after you graduate.

RESPONSIBILITY

Personal responsibility is key in school, work, and life. At school, you need to be responsible for managing your time, completing your work, and doing your best. As a health care professional, you will be responsible for all of those things and more—you'll be responsible for caring for patients, too.

Here are some things to keep in mind about your responsibilities at school and later in your career.

- You are responsible for your job—and *only* your job. It's great to help others when you can—you'll need the return favor some hectic day—but if others try to talk you into doing their work for them, politely refuse. Avoid adding tasks to your own. You may not be qualified to do them, or they may be someone else's responsibility.

- You are responsible for your time—manage it well. Be able to account for it.

- You are responsible for your things—make sure you have the materials and supplies you need to do your job. Make sure everything is where you need it.

- You are responsible for security and privacy. File sensitive patient information immediately, and only share it with your supervisor.

- You are responsible for being educated and informed— keep brushing up on your job skills. Read professional journals, talk with colleagues, and ask questions. Ask to sit in on specific procedures if you need improvement. Review your old textbooks and make sure you know what you're doing.

- You are responsible for your actions—avoid the urge to blame someone else in a situation where your actions are being examined. Take responsibility for your mistakes. It's much better than trying to lie or shift the blame. Your instructors, colleagues, and supervisors will respect you for being honest.

All of these skills are being honed now while you're in school. Time management, keeping track of your things, and making sure you really understand the material are the traits of a good student.

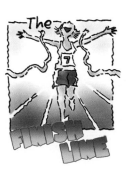

- Use the course documents provided by your instructor to find out what to expect in each course you take.

- Calculate your grades during the semester to make sure you're on target to meet your goals. Don't wait until it's too late for improvement!

- Organize your time by creating yearly, weekly, and daily schedules.

- Avoid procrastination by dividing large projects into several smaller tasks and setting realistic goals.

- Shape your honorable character now, and carry those good traits with you into your health care career.

Review Questions

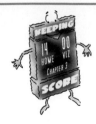

1. How can your syllabus help you be successful in a course?
2. What items do you need to put into your yearly schedule?
3. What challenges have you faced when it comes to honesty, accountability, or responsibility as a student?

Chapter Activities

Planning Exercise: Work as a group to create a long-term calendar for a student taking this course. Plan out the entire semester by referring to the syllabus or class schedule for information on:

- class times
- midterm and final exam dates
- due dates for papers and other projects
- deadlines for completing each phase of lengthy projects
- test dates
- the instructor's office hours
- deadlines for drop/add
- holidays and school vacations

WHAT'S MY SCORE?

Although some instructors provide periodic grade reports, there may be times when you need to figure out your grade on your own. Figuring out your grade means looking at what activities—tests, quizzes, homework, papers, etc.—you have to do to earn points and then seeing how much each activity counts toward your final grade. Your syllabus will tell you how many activities are required and how much each one counts toward your final grade.

He Shoots, He Scores!

Your instructor might assign a number of points or percentage values to each activity on the syllabus. Let's look at a grading system based on points first. If your instructor uses a point-based system, the easiest way to determine your grade is to convert the points to percentages. For example, if you take a test and receive a score of 40 out of 50 possible points (40/50), you can convert this score to a percentage to figure out your grade on the test. When figuring out percentages, remember to divide the number of points you received by the total number of possible points. A score of 40/50 equals 80%.

At any point during a semester or term, you also should be able to figure out your overall grade in a course. Let's say your syllabus lists the following information:

- five quizzes—worth 40 points each
- Test 1—worth 100 points
- Test 2—worth 200 points

So far, the class has taken one quiz and Test 1, for a total of 140 possible points (40 + 100 = 140). After adding up the points you received on the quiz and test, you find that you have a total of 120 out of 140 possible points (120/140). Based on this information, you can figure out your overall percentage grade.

120 ÷ 140 = 85.7%

If you keep track of your quiz and test scores (as well as any other graded activities) throughout the term, you'll be able to determine your overall grade in a course at any time. Knowing your grade in each course can help you gauge whether or not you're on target to meet your goals. Also, by keeping tabs on your grades, you can react early if they begin to slip. You may realize that you need to put in more study time, meet with your instructor, or visit the tutoring center. But if you wait until the end of the semester to figure out your overall grade in a course, it may be too late to improve it!

Batting Averages

Now let's look at a grading system based on *averages*. Suppose your instructor says that the average of six test grades will be your final grade in the course. By the middle of the term, the class has taken three tests. For example, if your test grades were 78%, 91%, and 95%, what would your overall grade be so far? Follow these simple steps to determine your average grade.

1. First, add your three test scores (78 + 91 + 95 = 264).
2. Then, divide the total by the number of tests you've taken so far (264 ÷ 3 = 88).

This means your grade in the course would be 88%. Much better than any professional baseball player's batting average!

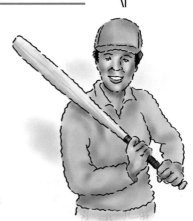

> To find your "batting average" in a course, just add up your scores and divide by the number of activities that have been assigned so far.

Weight Training

In some cases, each activity listed on a syllabus is *weighted*, or assigned a certain percentage of the final grade. This means some activities will affect your final grade more than others, as shown below.

- five quizzes—each is worth 10% of your final grade
- Test 1—worth 20% of your final grade
- Test 2—worth 30% of your final grade

Let's analyze these percentages. At first glance, it looks like the quizzes are not worth as much as Test 1 or Test 2. But look more closely; the syllabus says that *each* quiz is worth 10% of your final grade, which means:

5 quizzes × 10% = 50%

Because there are five quizzes, and each is worth 10%, the quizzes will make up 50%, or half, of your final grade. That's a big difference from 10%!

WHEN PROJECTS, PAPERS, AND HOMEWORK ARE IN PLAY

Many instructors also include activities, such as projects, papers, homework, and participation, in a student's final grade. Let's look at a scenario with several weighted activities.

- four quizzes—each is worth 5% of your final grade
- Test 1—worth 10% of your final grade
- Test 2—worth 20% of your final grade
- group project—worth 5% of your final grade
- homework—worth 5% of your final grade
- Attendance and participation make up the rest of your grade.

Now which is most important? You might think the quizzes or tests are more important to your final grade than your attendance and participation. Look more closely.

- Quizzes are 20% of your final grade (4 quizzes × 5% = 20%).
- The tests together equal 30% of your grade (10% + 20% = 30%).
- The group project plus homework equal 10% of your grade (5% + 5% = 10%).

That leaves 40% for your attendance and participation—the largest percentage of all!

But don't get confused and begin to think you can pass the course with low test and quiz scores because you're going to have perfect attendance. Think of it this way: you probably wouldn't make it as a professional basketball player if you can't dribble the ball, no matter how good your defensive play is!

Calculating Your Stats

So how do you figure out your grade in a course where the activities are weighted? Let's determine a student's grade based on the following syllabus information.

- quizzes—average of six quizzes is worth 15% of your final grade
- Test 1—worth 25% of your final grade
- Test 2—worth 60% of your final grade

Suppose a student averaged all of her quizzes for a score of 70%. On Test 1, her grade was 80%, and on Test 2, she received a score of 90%. How can we determine her final grade in the course if the activities are all weighted differently?

1. First, take all three scores and multiply each by the appropriate percentage, as listed on the syllabus. This will give each score the correct weight.

   quizzes—70(.15) = 10.5

   Test 1—80(.25) = 20

   Test 2—90(.60) = 54

2. Next, add the three products you came up with in step 1.

   10.5 + 20 + 54 = 84.5

3. The sum is the student's overall grade in the course: 84.5%.

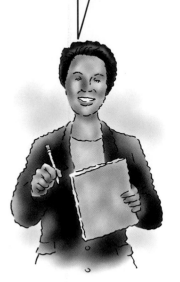

Keep track of your stats in each course by recording your scores when your instructor hands back graded assignments.

Grading Scales

It's no use knowing how many points you earned or what your grade averages were if you're unable to translate that information into a letter grade. Here's a sample grading scale from a syllabus.

97 – 100 = A+	76 – 79 = C+
94 – 96 = A	73 – 75 = C
90 – 93 = A–	70 – 72 = C–
86 – 89 = B+	66 – 69 = D+
83 – 85 = B	63 – 65 = D
80 – 82 = B–	60 – 62 = D–
	59 and under = F

For example, if a student received an overall grade of 84.5% in a course, that would translate to a B.

Many colleges use the 4.0 system to calculate student grade point averages (GPAs). To do this, they assign point values to each student's letter grades. Here's a sample chart based on the 4.0 system.

A+ – 4.3   C+ = 2.3

A = 4.0   C = 2.0

A– = 3.7   C– – 1.7

B+ = 3.3   D+ = 1.3

B = 3.0   D = 1.0

B– = 2.7   D– = 0.7

                  F = 0.0

Let's calculate the GPA of a student who has completed one semester of college. Suppose this student took four three-credit courses during his first semester. His overall grades were A, B+, A+, and C–. What would his GPA be?

1. First, list the point values assigned to each of the letter grades the student received.

    A   = 4.0

    B+ = 3.3

    A+ = 4.3

    C– = 1.7

2. Next, find the average of the four point values.

    4.0 + 3.3 + 4.3 + 1.7 = 13.3

    13.3 ÷ 4 = 3.325

3. The average is the student's GPA: 3.325 (which, rounded to the nearest decimal point, comes to 3.3).

    Keep in mind that the 4.0 system varies from school to school. For example, certain courses may be weighted more than others. You can talk to your academic advisor if you have questions about the system your school uses.

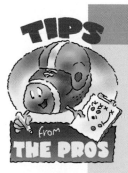

THE HOME STRETCH

Suppose you're in the home stretch—the term is almost over and you just have one more biology test to take. You'd really like to reach your goal of getting a B in the course, but you're not sure if that's possible. What grade would you have to get on the last test in order to get a B in the course?

1. First, look at the syllabus to see how much each graded activity is worth. For example, suppose your syllabus lists this information:

- five quizzes—average of five quizzes is worth 20% of your final grade
- Test 1—worth 30% of your final grade
- Test 2—worth 50% of your final grade

2. Next, list your scores for each activity. Let x stand for the score of your last test, since you haven't taken it yet. For the sake of this example, we'll use the following scores:

quizzes—70%

Test 1—75%

Test 2—x

3. Then, take all three scores and multiply each by the appropriate percentage, as listed on the syllabus. This will give each score the correct weight.

quizzes—70(.20) = 14

Test 1—75(.30) = 22.5

Test 2—x(.50) = .5x

4. Now, add the three products you came up with and make the sum equal to 80, as below. (This will be a basic algebraic equation used to find the value of x.) The value of x is the percent grade you will need to get on the test in order to receive a B (or at least 80%) in the course.

$14 + 22.5 + .5x = 80$

$36.5 + .5x = 80$

$36.5 + .5x - 36.5 = 80 - 36.5$

$.5x = 43.5$

$.5x \div .5 = 43.5 \div .5$

$x = 87$

5. And you have your answer! In order to receive a B in the course, you'd have to score at least 87% on the last test.

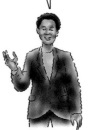

A simple equation can help you figure out how to achieve your goal grade in a course.

Grade Calculation Practice

At the midpoint in a semester, suppose a student has received the following scores:

- quizzes—8/10, 6/10, 9/10, 10/10
- homework assignments—5/5, 4/5, 3/5, 5/5

- research paper—139/150
- midterm exam—184/200

Based on the information above, calculate the following percentages (check your answers in the Appendix):

1. Assuming that each activity is weighted equally, what is the student's overall grade in the course so far?
2. What is the student's average quiz grade?
3. What is the student's average homework grade?
4. What percentage grade did the student receive on the research paper?
5. What percentage grade did the student receive on the midterm exam?

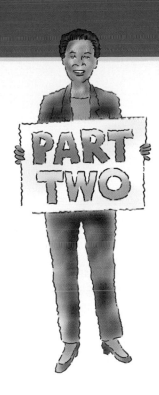

Sharpening Your Skills

Chapter 4

LEARNING—WHAT'S YOUR STYLE?

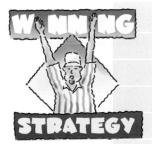

- Describe the brain's role in learning

- Recognize your learning style

- Develop a strategy for reading actively

- Create a note-taking outline

- Take effective notes in class

- Maximize your learning in the classroom

- Know the benefits of the Internet and e-mail

- Identify and describe several different types of electronic media

- Determine the difference between reliable and unreliable Web sites

- Conduct successful Internet searches

Did you know there are different styles of learning? For example, you might absorb information better when you see it (as in a chart) than when you hear it (as in a lecture). Some people learn better when they can "do" the material, as in a lab experiment. Your class is probably made up of students who have a variety of different learning styles. What works for one student might not work as well for the next.

This chapter discusses several major learning styles and how you can use your individual learning style, as well as other methods, to become a successful student.

Learning Styles

Your brain, and how it functions, is a contributing factor to the way you learn. By understanding how your brain works, you'll be able to identify your particular learning style. And by being aware of your learning style, you'll discover ways you can learn more efficiently.

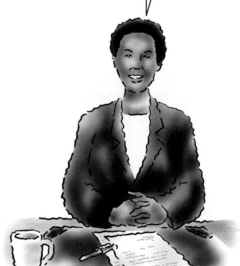

The way your brain works has an effect on how you learn.

THE BRAIN AND LEARNING

The human brain weighs about 3 pounds. Although small, this organ functions as the control center for the entire body. It determines how a person thinks, feels, and acts. The brain is where all learning takes place.

Your Hard-working Brain

It's true that people use only a percentage of the brain's full capability. Even so, the human brain is responsible for an amazing number of functions, including:

- breathing, temperature regulation, and other involuntary functions
- balance and equilibrium
- voluntary actions
- emotional reactions
- reasoning and thinking
- the ability to convert things you experience with your senses into recognizable images, sounds, feelings, smells, or tastes

Brain Zones

The three main areas of the brain include:

- the brain stem
- the cerebellum
- the cerebrum (See *The Human Brain*)

THE HUMAN BRAIN

The three main areas of the brain all have different roles in the learning process:

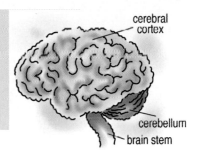

- Brain stem: connects the brain to the spinal cord and controls basic functions
- Cerebellum: controls basic functions, such as balance and coordination
- Cerebral cortex: controls high-level functions and voluntary muscle movements

Star Players: The Brain Stem and Cerebellum

The different areas of the brain all work together. However, each area is responsible for controlling certain functions. For example, the brain stem and cerebellum, located nearest the spinal cord, control basic functions. These areas of your brain determine your body's ability to maintain muscle tone. They also regulate involuntary actions, such as your heartbeat and breathing.

Team Captain: The Cerebrum

The cerebrum, the largest portion of the brain, contains the cerebral cortex. The cerebral cortex is very complex. It controls many high-level functions of the mind, such as sight and conscious thought. It also controls the body's voluntary muscle movements.

The brain's cortex is divided into two hemispheres. Different types of thought processes begin in each hemisphere.

- The left hemisphere is responsible for controlling language and logical thinking. In terms of physical movement, the left hemisphere controls the right side of the body.

- The right hemisphere, however, controls nonverbal processes, such as intuitive thinking and imagination. It manages movement of the left side of the body.

You may have heard the expressions "left-brained" and "right-brained." If a person is an artistic daydreamer, he may be considered "right-brained." A mathematician, on the other hand, may be considered "left-brained." One hemisphere of their brains may be more dominant, making certain tasks easier than others. This doesn't mean those individuals only use a single hemisphere of their brains. On the contrary, the left and right hemispheres of the brain are always active. Whether your personality is more logical or creative, you can use both sides of your brain. When it comes to learning, knowing your brain's strengths and weaknesses is helpful.

LEFT-BRAIN V. RIGHT-BRAIN

You may be a musician with an ear for rhythm or a math whiz with an eye for sequential order. In either case, both hemispheres of your brain are available to help you learn. By recognizing which hemisphere of your brain is stronger, you'll become aware of the kinds of tasks that require your brain to work slightly harder. The illustration below lists the major "left-brain" and "right-brain" reasoning tasks.

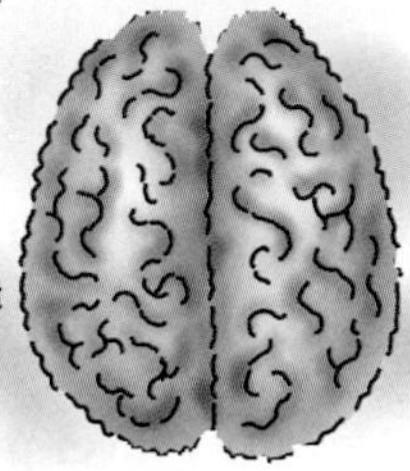

Left Hemisphere
- language and word use
- logic, reason, and analysis
- numbers and math
- rational thought
- sequence and order

Right Hemisphere
- artistic perception
- creativity
- intuitive thought
- music and rhythm
- imagination and abstract thought
- daydreaming and reflection
- random thought

On a Cellular Level

There are two main types of brain cells. They are:

- *glial cells.* These cells are the brain's supporting structures.
- *neurons.* These cells receive and send messages to one another in the form of electrochemical nerve impulses. Neurons play a role in complex functions of the mind and body, such as learning, motion, and sensations.

Good News Travels Fast!

News travels fast in the human brain. For example, an electrical signal travels from one neuron to the next at a rate of 200 miles per hour (100 meters per second)! These electric signals move from one neuron to another through a network of dendrites and axons.

The steps below trace the path of an electrical signal from one neuron to the next.

1. The electrical signal travels down the axon.
2. The axon releases neurotransmitters (chemicals).
3. The neurotransmitters travel across the synaptic gap and are received by the dendrites of the next neuron.
4. The next neuron absorbs the neurotransmitters.
5. The neurotransmitters change the second neuron's electrical state.
6. A new electrical pulse is produced by the second neuron.

Making Connections

Each infant is born with a complete set of neurons. As a child learns, those neurons develop connections between themselves. Every time sensory cells are stimulated by outside forces, nerve impulses travel from one neuron to the next.

Every time you learn something new, the neurons in your brain begin sending messages in a certain pattern. If stimulation is repeated, it becomes easier for the same nerve impulses to travel from one neuron to the next. This is because patterns begin to form and the neurons involved gain better connections between themselves. Your neurons "learn" these patterns and develop faster ways of communicating with each other.

Losing Ground

Learning new information causes the number of connections between your neurons to increase. Unfortunately, it's a two-way street. As soon as you stop learning new things, some of those connections begin to disappear. The solution to the problem is continued learning. You can rebuild those lost connections by relearning things you've forgotten.

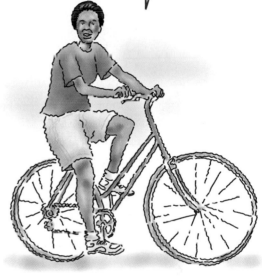

Learning new things, such as how to ride a bike, develops connections between your neurons. The more you practice something, the stronger those connections become.

Keeping Your Brain Healthy

A healthy body translates to a healthy mind. By taking care of your body, you'll be taking care of your brain too. And if you treat your brain right, you'll become a better learner.

You're probably aware that your diet has an impact on your physical performance. A doughnut in the morning won't give you lasting energy. But a healthy breakfast, such as a bowl of oatmeal and a cup of yogurt, will give you energy. Believe it or not, the food you eat and the fluids you drink affect how you learn as well. Diet has been linked to mood, behavior, and mental performance. For example, substances called electrolytes actually speed your thought processes. These substances work as conductors in the brain. Electrolytes help conduct the electrical currents that travel from one neuron to the next. Put simply, they help your brain think faster and work more efficiently.

Chapter 1 discussed healthy eating as a way to help your body cope with stress. Another reason to have a well-balanced diet is that it can enhance your ability to learn.

Brain Food

The key to keeping your body and mind in top working condition is to have a well-balanced diet. Electrolytes, such as potassium, calcium, and magnesium, improve your physical and mental performance. Consider incorporating foods that contain these nutrients into your healthy eating plan.

Good sources of potassium include:

- fish, such as salmon, cod, flounder, and sardines
- vegetables, such as broccoli, peas, lima beans, tomatoes, and potatoes (with their skins)
- leafy green vegetables, such as spinach and parsley
- citrus fruits
- other fruits, such as bananas, apples, and dried apricots

Good sources of calcium include:

- milk
- yogurt
- cheese
- soybeans
- some vegetables, such as collard greens and spinach

Good sources of magnesium include:

- some fish, such as halibut
- dry roasted nuts, such as almonds, cashews, and peanuts
- soybeans
- spinach
- whole grains
- potatoes (with their skins)

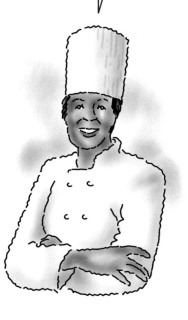

Today's specials are a treat for the brain as well as the palate—a well-balanced diet with a side of electrolytes!

Eating Smart

Eating right can be fairly simple. Just remember these basic guidelines.

- Make sure you include different types of food in your diet each day, such as vegetables, fruit, grains, and low-fat proteins.
- Check nutrition labels and look for foods low in saturated fat and cholesterol.
- Try to limit your intake of sugar, salt, and oils.
- Eat or drink caffeinated food or beverages in moderation.

- Drink plenty of water and avoid drinking too much alcohol.
- Balance the number of calories you eat each day with the amount of physical activity you do.

WHAT'S YOUR STYLE?

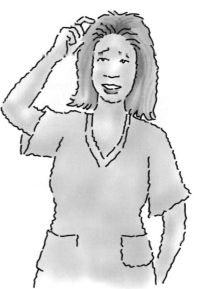

What's my learning style?

Now that we have looked at how the brain functions, let's focus on learning styles. Five major learning styles are:

- visual
- auditory
- kinesthetic
- global
- detail

Just as one hemisphere of your brain might be more dominant than the other, it's likely that you prefer one particular learning style to the rest. Use this knowledge to your advantage. Being aware of your learning strengths can help you improve your studying and test-taking skills. You'll also be better equipped to compensate for your weaknesses. By making your learning style work for you, you'll get more out of your courses. As an added benefit, you just might begin to enjoy the learning process.

The Eyes Have It

Visual learners prefer to read about things or watch demonstrations. If you're a visual learner, seek out all kinds of visual materials. These include:

- textbooks
- demonstrations (in class or on video)
- handouts from your instructors
- information on the Internet
- lecture notes
- articles in magazines, newspapers, and professional journals

Sounds Good to Me

Auditory learners gain the most information when they hear about things. If you learn best by listening, think of where you can find auditory information. Resources that may be helpful to you include:

- class discussions
- class lectures
- question-and-answer sessions
- giving speeches
- reading aloud
- study groups
- recorded lectures or speeches (video or online)

Jump Right In

Kinesthetic learners prefer to learn by doing. If it's easier for you to grasp information after putting it to use by actively doing something, you're a kinesthetic learner. To enhance your learning opportunities:

- Seek out workshops and skills labs.
- Volunteer to perform in-class demonstrations.
- Attend field trips.
- Help out with group projects.
- Seek out internships or volunteer work in your field.
- Offer to tutor a classmate.

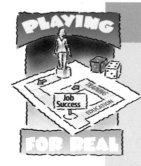

BEING A KINESTHETIC LEARNER

Hi, my name is Marcela and I'm training to become a surgical technician. I used to have a hard time learning new information. I'd read something and it wouldn't sink in. Or I'd sit and listen to a lecture only to feel like I wasn't getting it. I thought maybe I wasn't cut out for school.

That all changed when I took my first skills lab. All of a sudden, it's like a light bulb went on in my head! When I had a chance to demonstrate my skills, I actually understood and remembered the procedures.

Now that I know I'm a kinesthetic learner, I look for other ways to help me learn, in addition to reading my textbooks and going to classes. I attend workshops, go on field trips, and get plenty of hands-on experience volunteering at a local hospital.

Going Global

Global learners excel when they think about the "big picture." If you're a global learner, you may find that you enjoy learning how concepts are related to one another. Your favorite instructor may be one who gives plenty of analogies to show how the information is connected. Or you may prefer a class where the instructor lays out certain facts and helps students make conclusions about the material. If this is the case, try using the following tips to get the most out of your courses.

- Summarize your lecture notes and draw conclusions about the material.
- Sketch diagrams to show how different ideas come together to form the "big picture."
- Come up with questions about the topics covered in class.

It's All in the Details

Detail learners prefer to learn new information in a logical pattern. For example, many people have had the experience of purchasing items labeled "some assembly required." If you're prone to looking at instruction manuals and following directions closely—as opposed to jumping right in and fitting random pieces together—you're probably a detail learner.

If you're a detail learner, you may do best in a class where the instructor follows a strict outline. But regardless of your instructor's teaching style, there are ways you can use your strengths to your advantage.

- Summarize your lecture notes with bulleted points.
- Draw diagrams to relate small pieces of information (details) to larger themes or ideas.
- Create a to-do list for yourself before you sit down to study.
- Write down questions as they come to mind during lectures or while reading.
- Think of examples you can use to illustrate particular details.

Preparing for Class—The Need to Read

The relationship between a class of students and their instructor is comparable to the relationship between a team of athletes and their coach. Athletes must train on their own to master the basics of their sport. That way, they're prepared to refine their skills and learn about the nuances of the game when they meet with their coach. Similarly, when students work on their own to prepare for class, they become better equipped to understand and remember information from their instructor's lectures.

Even if you attend every lecture and participate in all classroom activities, you still need to prepare for class and read your course material. Reading is assigned by your instructor in an effort to help you understand concepts more fully.

For the visual learners out there, you're in luck. In most courses, over 75% of the information you receive will be in the form of printed materials. This means reading is an important part of preparing for class. If you learn best by reading, here's your opportunity to take advantage of your learning strengths and put them to good use.

If you don't happen to be a visual learner, be encouraged! Regardless of your particular learning style, all students can use the same methods to develop better reading skills and improve comprehension. Ways you can get more out of reading include:

- skimming for main ideas
- using active reading techniques
- reading chapter summaries to check your comprehension

The information in the following sections will show you how to become a more successful reader. If you aren't a visual learner, you may have avoided reading in the past whenever possible. However, this is an example of a time when being aware of your weakness is the first step toward improving upon it. If you *are* a visual learner and you enjoy reading, the tips in this section will help you hone your preferred method of learning.

If these methods are used often enough, they'll become routine. Soon, you'll be able to read a chapter without consciously thinking about the different tasks involved in reading.

START BY SKIMMING

Before you begin reading a chapter, flip though the pages and skim the material first. Doing this will give you a chance to look at the general organization of the chapter and identify key points. The purpose of skimming is to get your brain in gear so you'll absorb more information during active reading. By taking the time to skim over the chapter first, you'll give your brain the time it needs to begin organizing information in your head. This means you'll be able to mentally file information as soon as you begin reading. Not only does skimming allow you to understand the material more quickly, it helps you to remember more of what you read.

When skimming a chapter, follow these steps:

1. Look at the illustrations, graphs, charts, and tables. Read any captions.

2. Read the chapter introduction (usually located in the first paragraph).

3. Read the section headings throughout the chapter.

4. Take note of emphasized words in bold or italics as you flip though the pages.

5. Read the chapter summary (usually located in the closing paragraph).

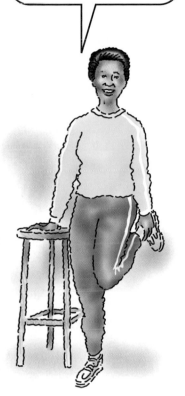

Skimming a chapter before reading it is like stretching your muscles before running a race. You need to make sure your brain is prepared to learn new information!

Graphic elements, such as charts and tables, illustrate important concepts covered in the chapter. Often, graphics provide snapshot views of the same information it may take several pages of text to explain. If you glance at each graphic element while skimming a chapter, you'll give yourself a quick preview of the material.

Build a Solid Foundation

When preparing to read a difficult chapter, make sure you first have some background knowledge of the topics covered. When you have a good foundation of knowledge on which to build, you'll have an easier time understanding complex new ideas.

For example, suppose a dental assistant and an experienced radiology technician both read a passage on using contrast media in certain x-ray procedures. Which individual would be able to comprehend the material more quickly and easily? Although both people may have had some experience taking x-rays, the radiology technician is likely to have a better foundation of knowledge. The technician's background and experience would give him an advantage over the dental assistant, who wouldn't have had the opportunity of working with contrast media. Even the technician's familiarity with the vocabulary used to describe such procedures would make it easier for him to read and understand the text.

As a student, how can you expand your foundation of knowledge? One way to give yourself some background information is to read a newspaper or magazine article on the topic. Another way to prepare for reading a difficult chapter would be to attend a lecture or seminar on a related topic. At the very least, you'd become familiar with the vocabulary used in the chapter. By the time you sat down to read your textbook, you would be able to focus your energy on trying to understand the concepts presented, as opposed to trying to figure out what specific words meant.

Take a Look at the Structure

Along with relating new information to your background knowledge, another tactic for skimming text is looking at how the chapter is organized. The chapter text may be structured in several different ways:

- *Subject development or definition structure.* These paragraphs present a single concept and then list supporting details. Introductory paragraphs usually are structured this way.

- *Sequence structure.* These paragraphs usually include signal words, such as *first, second, next, then, and finally.* The information in these paragraphs is presented in sequential order. Numbered lists also fall into this category.

- *Compare and contrast structure.* These paragraphs discuss how two or more concepts are alike and different. Words that signal comparisons include *both, similarly, too,* and *also.* Contrasting statements may include the signal words *yet, but, however,* or *on the other hand.*

- *Cause and effect structure.* These paragraphs often include signal words or phrases, such as *cause, effect, due to, in order to, resulting from,* and *therefore.* These paragraphs explain how one idea or event results from another idea or event.

Once you know how the text is organized, you'll be able to pinpoint the most important information. This will provide you with focus when the time comes to read the full chapter.

READY, SET, READ!

After you've skimmed the chapter, you can begin reading actively. But note that active reading goes beyond simply recognizing the words on each page. It includes using other tactics to aid your comprehension. In order to make sure you're reading actively, try putting some of the following tips into practice.

- Read aloud.

- Take notes or draw graphics as you read.

- Write down any questions you have about confusing concepts or ideas.

- Think about how information in the chapter relates to important points outlined in the table of contents (or outlined at the beginning of the chapter).

- Make a note of any difficult sections you'd like to read a second time.

Stay Focused

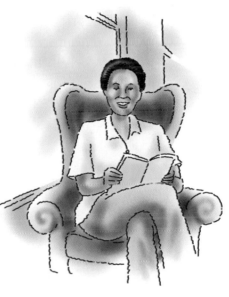

Help yourself avoid distractions by finding a quiet place to read.

Active reading requires concentration. Here are some basic guidelines to help you stay focused. (Chapter 6 provides additional study tips.)

- Read during the time of day you are most alert.
- Avoid trying to read too much at one time. When you start to feel your mind wandering, take a 5 minute break.
- Find a quiet place to read. Avoid distractions, such as watching TV or listening to loud music.
- Sit in a comfortable (but not too comfortable!) chair in order to stay awake and alert while reading.
- Supply yourself with a healthy snack and water to avoid getting distracted by being hungry or thirsty.

Post-Game Highlights

As you actively read each chapter, high-light important ideas or mark them with sticky notes. You can also make notes right in the margins. Just be careful not to mark too much text. If 90% of the material on every page is highlighted, it doesn't truly show which ideas are most important. But a chapter that is highlighted correctly is an excellent study tool. Being able to locate key ideas quickly will help you study more efficiently.

When deciding which text to highlight, think about what should be considered truly "important" material. Here are some hints.

- It's a good idea to highlight any information your instructor stresses in class. If your instructor considers a particular topic important, chances are that topic may appear on a test or quiz.
- It's also wise to highlight portions of text that answer any questions you came up with while skimming the chapter.
- Another rule of thumb is to look for and highlight topic sentences. These sentences discuss the main idea(s) in each paragraph.

Highlighting can help you find important information later, but keep in mind that it doesn't actually help you learn the material. To learn the information, spend a few extra minutes summarizing the text you highlighted in your own words. If you prefer, create a chart or diagram instead to illustrate key points. This helps you process the information and commit it to memory.

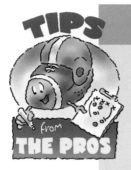

BRIGHT IDEA: HIGHLIGHTING TEXT

By highlighting text and making notes in the margins of your textbook, you'll remember more of what you read. You'll also be able to locate key ideas later when studying for the next test or quiz. Keep these tips in mind as you read.

- Read the entire paragraph or section before highlighting any portion of it.
- Highlight portions of text that answer any questions you thought of while skimming the chapter.
- Look for items presented in sequential order and number them accordingly.
- Highlight key terms, names, dates, and places.
- Summarize main ideas in the margins.
- Insert a question mark next to confusing paragraphs or sentences. Write any questions or comments you may have in the margins.
- Mark any information your instructor considers important with a star or exclamation point.
- Highlight important information in the table of contents or create a list of the most important topics.

Make It Personal

Another way to make sure you're reading actively is to connect with the material on a personal level. By making the information more personal, you'll have an easier time remembering it. You can do this by:

- *Making associations*. For example, you might be able to remember an important date by associating it with the birthday of someone you know. (Chapter 6 discusses associations in more detail.)

- *Having an emotional response to the material*. Reacting to the information you read will make it more memorable.

- *Drawing pictures to illustrate different concepts*. A picture might be easier to remember than a paragraph of text.

Be Critical

During active reading, it's important to be a critical reader. Now is the time to analyze the text and question the author. By asking questions about the text, you'll begin to think critically about the material. As a result, you'll improve your comprehension and possibly remember more of the information. Ask yourself:

- How would I apply this information if I were caring for a patient?

- How is this material related to what I've studied in the past?

- How does this information measure up to the information in other sources I've read? Does it support or contradict what I already know about the topic?

- Are there any inconsistencies?

- Does the author present an objective view of the material? Is the information based on assumptions, facts, experiences, or opinions?

- Do I agree with the author? Why or why not?

- On which topic would I like more information?

Know the Lingo

Reading actively also involves making sure you understand the vocabulary used to describe new concepts. This means you must determine the meaning of an unfamiliar word before continuing your reading. In scientific texts especially, it's important to know the meaning of the technical terms used. Knowing the vocabulary makes your job of understanding the material much easier. For example, suppose you were required to read a passage discussing what happens to the body during a myocardial infarction. Knowing that *myocardial infarction* is the technical term for "heart attack" would help you understand the passage more readily.

When you notice an unfamiliar word, first try to figure out its meaning from its context clues. Context clues can include other words or sentences that provide hints about the word's meaning. They also can include root words, prefixes, and suffixes. If you're unable to determine the word's meaning from its context clues, look it up in a dictionary or glossary. Then, make a note of the definition and pronunciation in the margin of your textbook or in your notes. If the word appears once in the chapter, it may appear again.

When skimming a chapter, you may notice many unfamiliar words. It may be helpful to look up all the definitions before you begin actively reading the text.

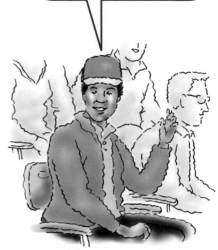

A baseball game makes a lot more sense if you're familiar with the lingo. The same is true for reading scientific texts. If you don't know a word, look it up!

Read Chapter Summaries

In most textbooks, each chapter is formatted similarly. Therefore, the chapter summary always should appear in roughly the same place. It usually appears toward the end of the chapter in the form of a summary paragraph, bulleted statements, or review questions.

One of the last steps in active reading is reviewing the chapter summary. Read the chapter summary and refer back to the table of contents to make sure you understood the key points of the chapter. If there are sections you didn't understand, reread them or make a note to ask your instructor for clarification.

When rereading, try using a different method than you used during your first active reading of the chapter. You could adjust the speed of your reading by reading a particular section more slowly, for example. Reading aloud is another method. When rereading text, make an effort to understand each sentence before continuing. Think about how each new concept you come across relates to other information in the chapter.

Effective Note-taking

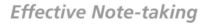

Chapter 2 gave several reasons why note-taking is important. Notes provide you with study points when the time comes to prepare for tests and quizzes. They also help you stay focused during class. This section discusses several methods all students can use to take effective notes.

START BEFORE CLASS

Review your textbook and create a note-taking outline before each lecture. This familiarizes you with the material and helps to organize your notes. By locating key terms and main ideas beforehand, you'll provide yourself with a basic outline to follow and fill in during the lecture. In essence, your note-taking outline is your "road map" for the lecture. By using it, there's less chance of getting lost!

To help you determine which terms and concepts to include in your outline, follow these steps:

1. Look at the general layout of the chapter. Make a mental note of each section's length—longer sections will need more space in your outline.

2. Read the introductory paragraph. The first paragraph in a chapter often lists main ideas.

3. Review any graphs, charts, or diagrams.

4. Search for any bold or italic words. If a word or phrase is emphasized in the chapter, it should be included in your outline.

5. Read the closing paragraph. The last paragraph in a chapter usually summarizes important information and draws conclusions.

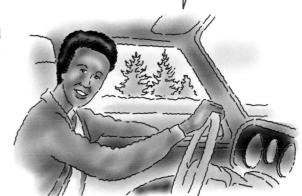

During the lecture, fill in any gaps left in your outline. Add to it by including information from the lecture that is not provided by your textbook.

TAKE NOTES IN CLASS

It may seem as if some students were born with the ability to take good notes. But note-taking is a learned skill! You can learn how to take effective notes by using the following tips.

- Use shorthand.
- Make sure your notes contain personal applications.
- Avoid tape recording lectures.
- Use a note-taking strategy that fits your style of learning and your instructor's style of teaching.
- Organize your notes.

Shorthand Helps You Keep Up the Pace

Develop your own shorthand for note-taking. By abbreviating words and using symbols, you'll be able to keep up with a fast-paced lecture. To improve your speed in taking notes:

- Abbreviate commonly used words. For example, the abbreviation pt. can be used for the word *patient*. You can make up your own abbreviations. Just remember to use them consistently.

- Develop shorthand symbols for other common words. For example, the symbol → means "leads to" or "causes."

- Leave out conjunctions (*or, and, but*) and prepositions (*of, in, for, on, to, with,* etc.) if they aren't needed to understand the idea.

- Take a moment to think before you jot down a note. This helps you focus on one thought and write it down quickly.

- Avoid copying text directly out of the textbook. Instead, highlight the text in your book and refer to the appropriate page number in your notes.

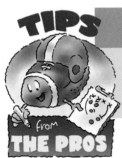

USE SYMBOLS + ABBR.

Below are some common note-taking abbreviations and symbols. Speed your note-taking by using these shortcuts or coming up with your own.

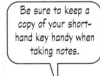

Be sure to keep a copy of your shorthand key handy when taking notes.

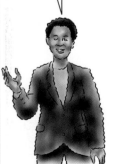

Abbreviations		Symbols	
abt	about	®	right
b/c	because	Ⓛ	left
dx	diagnose or diagnosis	↑	increase, increased, or increasing
e.g.	for example	↓	decrease, decreased, or decreasing
ha	headache	→	leads to or causes
hx	history	>	more than
imp	important	<	less than
incl	including	Δ	change
pt.	patient	~	about, approximately
px	physical	+	and, in addition
rx	treat or treatment	#	pounds or number
se	side effects	*	important or stressed by instructor
s/s	signs and symptoms	p̄	after
w/	with	ā	before
w/o	without	-	negative
		c̄	with
		s̄	without

Apply It!

Be sure to include personal applications in your notes. Write down cues to help you link new information to your previous knowledge. This not only helps you maintain active listening, it will also help you study the material later.

Using someone else's lecture notes should be a last resort. Copying notes doesn't allow you to analyze the material. For this reason, borrow notes only on the rare occasions when you are unable to attend a class. You'll have an easier time learning the information if you're present for each lecture and take notes yourself.

Pen and Paper Are Better

Although it may seem like a wise idea, tape-recording lectures isn't the most efficient way to learn or study new material. Some of the problems with recording are:

- It increases your review/study time. It only takes a few minutes to read through your lecture notes for the day. However, listening to the entire lecture all over again takes much longer.

- A tape recording doesn't include diagrams or other important information the instructor writes on the chalkboard during a lecture.

- Even your best intentions can be thwarted by technical difficulties. Dead batteries or a poor quality recording can cause you to miss out on important information from the lecture.

- Not all instructors allow students to record their lectures. If you must use a tape recorder, ask your instructor before class.

There is one, and only one, instance when tape recording might be your best option. If you ever have to miss a class, it may be helpful to have a classmate tape the lecture. In this case, listening to the lecture on tape and taking your own notes might be more beneficial than simply copying someone else's notes.

Note-taking—What's Your Style?

Develop a note-taking style that works best for you. Below are some suggestions for personalizing your method of note-taking:

- Remember how to read your own shorthand by creating a key to keep in your notebook.

- Copy down information and diagrams that your instructor writes on the chalkboard.

- Write neatly so you'll be able to use your notes when studying for quizzes and tests.
- Leave space in your notes that you can fill in later with information from your textbook.
- Read over your notes after class and make any necessary corrections.
- Separate groups of ideas by skipping a line in your notes.
- Use a color-coding system to mark groups of ideas or to emphasize important terms and concepts.

Your note-taking style also should work well with how your instructor lectures. Your notes can be formatted in several different ways. Keep your instructor's teaching style in mind when choosing a format for your lecture notes.

- *Outline.* This format works well with instructors who follow strict outlines and give very organized lectures.
- *Asymmetrical columns.* If your instructor frequently gives reminders ("Remember this for the test on Tuesday") or refers to your textbook during lectures ("Let's look at page 52"), this format may work best for you.
- *Compare/contrast.* This format works well with an instructor who often discusses two separate topics at the same time in an effort to show how the topics are alike and different.
- *Concept map.* This format works well with instructors who provide many anecdotes or examples of a single main idea, but who don't necessarily follow a strict outline.

Another formatting tip is to leave space (2 inches or so) at the bottom of each page for a brief summary. Reviewing your notes and summarizing each page after class helps you process the information.

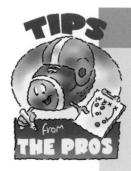

TIPS from THE PROS

FORMATTING YOUR NOTES

Below are a few examples of different note-taking formats.
Outline: This format helps you organize the information.

Asymmetrical Columns: This format allows plenty of room for you to write comments, questions, or reminders next to your lecture notes.

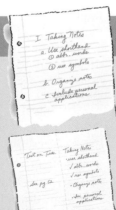

Compare/Contrast: This format gives you an easy way of looking at how two different concepts are alike and different.

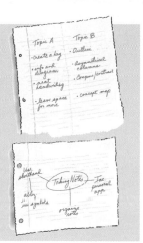

Concept Map: This format allows you to show how several different anecdotes or examples are connected to a single main idea.

A Cinematic Experience

You may need to use a slightly different approach when taking notes on a film, television segment, or slide presentation shown during class. Although the classroom may be dark, these are not good times to tune out or doze off!

If the room is too dark for you to take notes during a film, pay close attention and jot down a brief summary or a few key points after class. If the film or TV show moves too quickly and doesn't allow you enough time to take effective notes, consider watching it again. Often, instructors place these types of presentations on reserve in the campus library. Watching the film or looking at the slides a second time will give you a chance to write down any important information you missed during class.

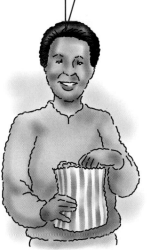

When your instructor shows a film during class, it's not leisure time! Take notes to get the most out of it.

Finding a Happy Medium

The amount of notes you take determines their effectiveness. Taking too few notes means you won't have enough material to jog your memory later. However, taking too many notes during class won't allow you any time to think about and process the information. So how do you know when enough is enough?

If your notes resemble a brief, disorganized list of facts, you're probably taking too few. In this case, focus on noting how those facts relate to one another. On the other hand, if your pen never leaves the page during class, you might be taking too many notes. Instead, work on writing down only the most important information. By finding a happy medium, your notes will become more effective.

A NOTE AFTER CLASS

The most important thing to remember about your notes is to review them. Try to look over your notes within 24 hours after class. It's easier to make corrections and add to your notes while the lecture is still fresh in your mind. Reviewing your notes soon after you take them also helps you commit the information to memory.

GETTING ORGANIZED

As you read in Chapters 2 and 3, organization is critical to your success as a student. It also makes a difference in the effectiveness of your notes. Your lecture notes can be an excellent study tool, but not if they're in a disorganized jumble of papers. Take the time, either during or after class, to organize your notes. You'll thank yourself later!

Getting the Most out of Class

Taking notes isn't the only way to increase learning in the classroom. You'll need to do things in addition to taking notes in order to increase your learning potential. Get the most out of class by focusing on:

- information presented in handouts
- key terms or ideas the instructor writes on the chalkboard
- concepts the instructor emphasizes during the lecture
- any questions raised by classmates and your instructor's responses to those questions
- your own opinions and thoughts about material presented by your instructor
- material that isn't covered in the textbook
- your instructor's teaching style
- your instructor's introductory and summary statements (given at the beginning and end of each lecture)

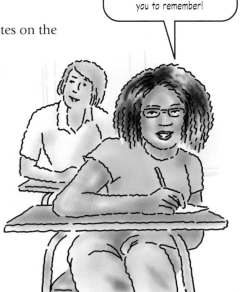

Knowing your personal learning style can give you an advantage in the classroom. Being aware of *how* you learn can help you increase the amount of information you understand and remember. By using a variety of learning techniques, you can accommodate your learning style. As a result, not only will you begin to perform better academically, you'll have better communication with your instructors.

BE AN ACTIVE LISTENER

One way to get more out of class is to be an active listener. Instead of sitting back and relaxing while your instructor lectures, try to keep your mind engaged. Make an effort to listen actively. To better understand the material, think of questions to ask the instructor. You can write your questions in the margins of your notes and refer back to them at the end of the lecture. If your instructor offers to answer any questions toward the end of class, ask then. If not, look up the answers on your own after class.

There may be times, however, when you'll have a question that can't wait until the end of the lecture. If you feel that your instructor is moving too quickly, politely interrupt and ask her to repeat or clarify a specific point. But keep in mind that you should do so only when you have prepared for the class properly beforehand.

At Breakneck Speeds

What happens if the instructor is moving too quickly? If you're prepared for class and keeping up with your reading and still can't keep up with the lecture, you should speak up! When doing this, be specific. Avoid interrupting with a vague statement such as, "I don't understand." This kind of statement implies that you didn't prepare for class. Also, it may be frustrating to your instructor because it doesn't indicate what information you need her to explain more fully. Instead, show your instructor what part of the material you *did* understand by summarizing it in your own words. Then, ask a specific question. For example, you could say, "I understand that sterile technique means doing things to prevent contamination, like wearing sterile gloves and using sterile instruments. But could you explain the difference between sterile technique and aseptic technique? Are they the same?"

Occasionally, you may feel like the only student in the class who isn't able to keep up. You're not alone—many students have felt this way at one point or another. If this is the case, it's probably because the other students in the class have a greater foundation of knowledge. They may have taken prerequisite courses that you haven't. If this happens, try not to get discouraged or give up following along with the lecture. Instead, make an effort to listen more closely and continue taking notes, being careful to write down confusing terms or concepts. After class, look in your textbook or ask your instructor for clarification. This practice of writing down what you don't understand is also helpful if you meet regularly with a tutor. It gives you specific pieces of information to review.

At a Snail's Pace

Alternatively, you may encounter instructors who present material at a much slower pace. If you allow yourself to become bored during these classes, your mind will begin to wander. To stay focused on the material, there are several tricks you can use.

- Practice summarizing information in your head. By forcing your brain to think about putting ideas into your own words, you'll stay alert.

- Try to memorize definitions of key terms as your instructor goes over them. Instead of simply reading the definitions or hearing about them, you'll be committing them to memory for future reference.

- Predict what information your instructor will cover next. This causes you to consider how your instructor thinks. You will gain a better understanding of what your instructor expects students to know.

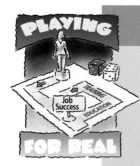

WHEN AN INSTRUCTOR MOVES TOO SLOWLY

My name is Sean. I'm going to school to become a medical coding specialist. For the most part, I've liked my classes, but I've had to take a few boring ones too. I had this one instructor who talked *so slowly* that I could hardly stay awake during class. Even when I'd bring a cup of coffee with me, I'd still find myself nodding off by the end of the lecture.

Then I found a solution. I realized it was a lot easier to stay awake if I had to think about the information and put it in my own words. So I'd just summarize what my instructor was saying in my head. It worked a lot better than caffeine!

COMMUNICATE WITH YOUR INSTRUCTOR

By staying engaged and asking questions about the lecture, you'll help your instructor clear up any misunderstandings about the material. Other students might be confused about the same concepts that are confusing to you. The instructor's answers to your questions may be helpful to your classmates as well.

Also, by speaking up in class, you'll let your instructor know how well you're grasping the material he's presenting. If an instructor feels that students are able to keep up with the pace of the class, he'll know his method of teaching is successful. If most students are unable to keep up, your instructor will be able to make adjustments or try presenting the material in a different way.

MAKE ADJUSTMENTS

Occasionally, you'll have to make your own adjustments for an instructor who doesn't present information clearly. In such cases, you may have to think of examples, draw conclusions, or apply new information on your own. To do these things, you'll need to maintain active listening.

Here are several tips you can use to make sure you keep listening actively.

- Remember your purpose for listening.
- Pay special attention to the beginning and end of the lecture, when your instructor might introduce and summarize key points.
- Take effective notes.
- Sit up straight to avoid feeling sleepy and to show your interest in the lecture.
- Make sure your eyes stay focused on the instructor.
- Ignore external and internal distractions by concentrating on the instructor's words.
- Analyze the material.
- Listen for main points.
- Make a note of words or concepts you don't understand so you can look them up after class.
- Adjust to the pace of the lecture.

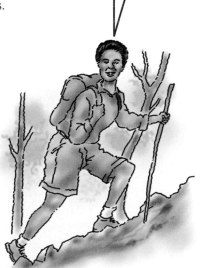

Trying to learn new material from a poor speaker might feel like you're climbing uphill. Show that you're up for the challenge by being an active listener!

Using Supplemental Material

Using supplemental material is another way to accommodate your personal learning style. If you have a hard time learning information from a lecture or a textbook, it's especially helpful to supplement your education. By having the same information presented to you in a variety of ways, you'll learn more and have better recall of important points. In contrast, you may use supplemental material as a way of finding out more about an interesting topic covered in one of your classes. Whatever your reason may be, making use of supplemental material gives you an advantage as a student.

Computers are a major source of supplemental material. Thus, having a working knowledge of computers is a necessity. You will use computers for many different purposes both during your time as a student and later in your professional career. As a student, you may use computers to:

- communicate with your classmates and instructors
- compose reports
- view information on textbook CDs
- run educational software programs
- perform research
- take courses online

As a health care professional, it's likely that you'll encounter computers on a daily basis. For example, if you work in a medical office one day, your office may use computers for such everyday tasks as scheduling appointments and billing patients.

If you aren't already, you will need to become computer literate, meaning you will need to understand the basic functions of computers and their software applications.

COMPUTER VOCABULARY

Becoming familiar with the technical terms used to describe computers and their functions will help you on your way to computer literacy.

Basic Parts

- *Hard drive.* A computer's hard drive stores electronic data.
- *Memory.* Memory indicates how much information a computer can process and store. The more memory a computer has, the more programs it can run and the more files it can store.

- *Modem*. A computer's modem gives it a way to send electronic data over telephone lines. Home computers that connect to the Internet with this type of modem have dial-up access. Some cell phone services now offer wireless Internet access. Other types of modems include cable (which allows data to be transmitted over a cable TV line) and DSL (which transmits data over a *digital subscriber line*).

- *Monitor*. A monitor is a screen that displays text and graphics. It looks similar to a TV screen.

- *Mouse*. A mouse is a small device that controls the cursor on the computer screen. It allows the user to "select" an object, open files and folders, and perform a variety of other tasks.

- *RAM*. RAM stands for *random-access memory*. It determines a computer's operating speed. It is measured in bytes (i.e., megabytes and gigabytes). The more RAM a computer has, the faster it can operate.

Outside the Computer

- *Floppy disk*. A floppy disk is a small (three and a half-inch wide) device that stores electronic data. Floppy disks are rarely used anymore.

- *CD-ROM*. A CD-ROM (*compact disk, read-only memory*) is a storage device. CD-ROMs can hold much more electronic data than floppy disks.

- *Jump drive*. A jump drive is a portable computer file storage device that uses flash memory. It's very small, lightweight, and connects to the computer's USB port.

- *Network*. Two or more computers linked together form a network. Computers within the same network can share information easily, without having to connect to the Internet. Many businesses and universities use networks.

- *Printer*. A printer is used to produce hard copies of text or images that appear on a computer screen. There are many different types of printers. They can print text in black or in color, while some color printers are designed to print graphics and photos as well as text.

- *Scanner*. A scanner "reads" text or graphics that appear on paper and converts them into an electronic or digital format the computer can use. Once a document or image has been scanned into a computer, the user can make changes to it.

COMPUTERS AND COMMUNICATION

Computers allow you to communicate at a distance—this process is called telecommunication. Two common forms of telecommunication include the Internet and e-mail.

Knowing the "language" of the computer world increases my computer literacy.

The Web

The Internet connects computers around the world. For this reason, it can be used as a communication tool. A large part of the Internet is the World Wide Web, or just "the Web." The Web allows businesses to communicate with each other and with consumers. For example, many businesses advertise their products or services on company Web sites. The Web has made it possible for small businesses to reach a wide market of consumers.

Students can use the Internet both in communicating with classmates and instructors and in conducting research. One method of communicating via the Internet would be through using online message boards (also called online discussion boards). These venues allow you to post questions or comments to your classmates and instructors. Some message boards are set up so students and instructors from different schools anywhere in the world can communicate with each other. Because their format encourages discussion, message boards can be a great source of supplemental material.

To access the Internet, your computer will need the proper software, the necessary hardware, and an Internet Service Provider (ISP). Internet-access software, also called a browser, includes such popular programs as Microsoft Internet Explorer, Mozilla Firefox, Netscape Navigator, and Avant Browser. Your computer will also need the necessary hardware—a modem or a wireless card. Lastly, your computer will need an ISP. An ISP is a company that provides you access to the Internet. ISPs provide local access from your computer to their computer network, and their network connects you to the Internet.

E-mail

E-mail is a shortened version of the term *electronic mail*. You probably are familiar with this form of telecommunication. E-mail allows people to send messages, documents, and digital pictures to anyone with Internet access. It helps people communicate with each other across the globe. Popular e-mail programs include Microsoft Outlook Express, Microsoft Entourage, Eudora, and Thunderbird.

You might be given a free e-mail account through your school. Remember to keep your school e-mail account separate from your personal account. This will help keep you and your school materials organized!

ELECTRONIC MEDIA

Electronic media are another type of supplemental material. Different forms of electronic media you may encounter as a student include textbook CDs and computer software.

Textbook CDs

Many textbooks come with instructional CDs. The CDs usually include practice exercises or supplementary information. Textbook CDs are designed to increase students' learning. Most present the same information as the textbook but in a different format. For example, some CDs may be interactive. This can be helpful to students who have a difficult time understanding the material as it's presented in the textbook. CDs also can be helpful to students looking for ways to improve their recall of information included in the textbook.

Software

Put simply, computer software refers to computer programs. In terms of supplemental material for students, there are many different kinds of software that you may find helpful. Types of software that are particularly beneficial to students include:

- practice exercises
- tutorials
- simulations
- assessments

Practice Makes Perfect

Some software provides practice exercises. These may be in the form of quizzes you can take or problems you can solve. The purpose of this type of software is to help students learn and remember facts and vocabulary. It also aids in your understanding of how different concepts are related. The more you practice, the more you'll be required to use your new knowledge. This increases your ability to remember and comprehend the material in your textbook.

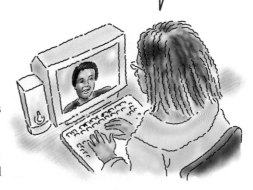

Students with full-time jobs or families may prefer to use tutorial software instead of taking extra time to meet with a tutor.

Your Own Private Tutor

If you find yourself lost even after attending lectures and getting clarification from your instructor, tutorial software can help. These programs are designed to teach concepts. Although they may include brief quizzes to assess your level of knowledge, the main focus of these programs is instruction. The material may be presented in several different formats, making use of text, images, and student responses.

Is This for Real?

Simulations are another type of educational software. Simulations are computerized versions of real-life experiences. They are interactive and often require decision-making on the part of the student. Health profession students can use these programs to learn or hone clinical skills. The beauty of simulations is that they are forgiving of mistakes made during the learning process. After all, it would be better to make a mistake while caring for a simulated patient than to make one while caring for an actual patient!

How Am I Doing?

Assessment software can be beneficial to students and instructors alike. On one hand, computerized testing helps students determine their level of knowledge. As a student, being aware of how much you know can help you set goals for yourself. It allows you to focus on what you have yet to learn. On the other hand, this type of software also can be helpful to instructors. Once they are able to determine their students' progress, they can adjust the curriculum appropriately.

INTERNET RESEARCH

Aside from being a communication tool, the Internet can help you perform research. By sitting down at a computer, you literally have access to a world of resources. The supplemental material you can find online far outweighs the volume of material stored in any library. The key is in determining which sources on the Web are reliable and which are not.

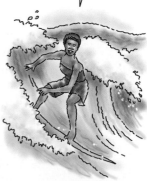

It's a good thing surfing the Web is a lot easier than this!

Web Sites

Web sites consist of one or more Web pages. When you are "surfing the Web," it means you are moving from one Web page to another. You're able to do this by clicking on hyperlinks, which usually look like graphics, buttons, or underlined words onscreen.

All Web sites have a "home page." This is the main page for the site. A home page usually includes text or graphics as well as links to additional pages within the site. Because there are billions of Web sites on the Internet, it's helpful to have an idea of how to search for particular information and which Web sites to trust. By following some simple guidelines, your online research will go more smoothly.

On the Corner of http:// and www

Each Web page has an address, otherwise known as a URL (universal resource locator). If you know a site's URL, you'll have no trouble locating it among the many other sites on the Web.

Web addresses, especially lengthy ones, might look confusing. But each address is made up of the same basic components. Below is an explanation of each component, based on the fictional Web address http://www.acmesportsequipment.com.

- *http://* These letters stand for hypertext transfer protocol. Most Web addresses start out this way.
- *www.* This acronym for World Wide Web appears in many, but not all, URLs.
- *acmesportsequipment* This portion of the Web address indicates the name of the site. In this example, the site is named for the Acme Sports Equipment Company.
- *.com* This portion of the URL is called the suffix. The suffix provides additional information about the site.

What's in a Name?

Usually, you can gather certain information about a Web site just by looking at the suffix of its URL. All U.S. sites are assigned a suffix according to the groups or individuals who own them. Here is a brief list of suffixes:

- *.com* This suffix usually indicates that a particular site is intended for commercial use. Most sites ending in .com are owned by businesses or individuals.
- *.edu* Web addresses ending in .edu indicate educational institutions (colleges and universities). If your school has a Web site, its URL probably ends in .edu.
- *.gov* This suffix indicates that a particular site is owned and operated by a government institution or agency.
- *.net* Web addresses ending in .net usually indicate ISPs.
- *.org* This suffix is used to indicate nonprofit organizations.

The Search Is On!

What happens if you don't know the URL of the site you're looking for? Or what if you prefer to search for several different Web sites that deal with a specific topic? This is where search engines come in.

For example, suppose you needed to locate information on how to perform cardiopulmonary resuscitation (CPR). You would go to a search engine on the Internet and enter keywords into the search box. For this particular search, *CPR* would be an appropriate keyword. The search engine would then compile a list of Web sites that may be relevant to your search. You would be able to view the results of your search and click on the links to Web sites that seemed applicable.

Below is a list of common search engines and their Web addresses.

When conducting online research, only use information from sites you can trust.

- About.com (www.about.com)
- Altavista (www.altavista. com)
- Ask.com (www.ask.com)
- Dogpile (www.dogpile.com)
- Excite (www.excite.com)
- Go.com (www.go.com)
- Google (www.google.com)
- Hotbot (www.hotbot.com)
- LookSmart (search.looksmart.com)
- Lycos (www.lycos.com)
- Snap (www.snap.com)
- Yahoo (www.yahoo.com)

The Reliability Test

Just because information has been posted on the Internet doesn't make it trustworthy. When performing research online, remember to be wary of unreliable Web sites. Here are some tips to use when trying to spot the difference between reliable and unreliable sites.

- Compare sources to verify information. If a statement posted on a Web site seems too outrageous to be true, check it against a source you trust.
- Beware of sites that seem biased or push a specific agenda. These sites may skew facts or give blatant misinformation.
- Pay attention to URL suffixes. Usually, you can assume that sites ending in .gov or .edu contain reliable information.

However, be wary of .edu sites that are owned by individual students at a university. These sites generally are not regulated for accuracy.

- As a general rule, the sites of well-known businesses or agencies that have good reputations tend to post reliable information.

- Be especially critical of information posted on sites owned by individuals or small, unknown organizations. The owners of these sites do not have the same accountability as reputable businesses or organizations.

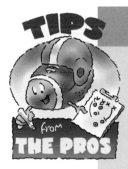

IMPROVE YOUR SEARCHING SKILLS

With so much information on the Web, it's sometimes tricky trying to locate the information you need. The following tips will help you perform better Internet searches.

Starting Your Search

- Avoid using words such as *a*, *an*, and *the* when entering keywords into a search bar. Most search engines ignore these words anyway.

- If you are looking for a specific phrase, enclose it in quotation marks. Most search engines recognize text contained within quotes as a single item. For example, if you needed to find information on heart disease in children, you would enter *"heart disease in children"* in the search bar.

- Be specific. Entering *diabetes education* in the search bar would give you fewer results to sort through than the more general search term *diabetes*.

- Avoid being overly specific. If your search returns very few results, broaden your search terms.

Keeping At It

- If your first search is unsuccessful, try rephrasing your keyword(s). In some ways, search engines are like indexes. Usually, when you can't find a particular word in an index, you can find what you need by looking up a related word. This principle works when conducting online searches as well.

- If you still can't find what you're looking for, try using a different search engine.

- If you continue experiencing problems, see if your search engine has an advanced search option. You may be able to enter more specific criteria for your search.

RELIABLE WEB SITES

Your instructor may be able to provide you with a more complete listing of reliable health professions Web sites. Here's a brief list to get you started.

Site Name	Address	Brief Summary
American Association of Medical Assistants	www.aama-ntl.org	Offers information for students and employers
American Dental Assistants Association	www.dentalassistant.org	Includes information on membership in the association, education, and employment
American Heart Association	www.americanheart.org	Includes information on continuing education and resources for professionals
American Red Cross	www.redcross.org	Offers health and safety information
American Society of Radiologic Technologists	www.asrt.org	Includes information on continuing education; provides links to online publications and an online learning center
HealthAnswers Education	www.healthanswers.com	Offers interactive training for individuals in the pharmaceutical and biotechnology industries
Lippincott Williams & Wilkins	www.lww.com	Publisher of allied health texts; provides health care news, continuing education information, and other resources
Massage Therapy Foundation	www.massagetherapyfoundation.org	Provides resources for students, including a massage therapy research database
MayoClinic.com	www.mayoclinic.com	Provides health information from the scientists and doctors at the Mayo Clinic
National Institutes of Health	www.nih.gov	Government-sponsored site; functions as the home page for all other NIH sites, such as the National Cancer Institute, National Institute on Aging, and others
WebMD	www.webmd.com	Offers health information and links to articles on health-related issues; provides online discussion boards

ONLINE INSTRUCTION

Yet another way to supplement your education is through online instruction. Courses taught online can include most of the elements from traditional classes, such as instructor-led presentations, question and answer sessions, assignments, and tests.

More schools are beginning to offer online courses. A major benefit of online courses is the flexibility they offer students, especially students who continue to work while going to school. Being able to take a course while at home can simplify lots of things, and save time and money. Just the time saved by not commuting back and forth to class makes it a very attractive alternative!

Just remember to keep your learning style in mind when considering an online course. For example, a student who is an auditory learner may struggle in an online course that requires a lot of extra reading. However, a visual learner may thrive in such a course. Choose an online course that provides instruction in a format that works for you.

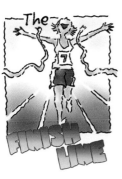

- Your brain plays a role in determining your particular learning style.

- Play to your strengths by recognizing your learning style and being aware of how to enhance it.

- Reading is a two-part process that includes skimming and active reading.

- Give yourself a road map to follow during class by creating a note-taking outline.

- Develop a note-taking style that works for you. Keep your instructor's lecturing style in mind when deciding how to format your notes.

- Use supplemental material to increase your learning. Resources, such as textbook CDs, educational software, the Internet, and online instruction, can provide benefits beyond the classroom.

- Determine the difference between reliable and unreliable Web sites by looking at the site name and evaluating the information posted on the site. Be critical!

- Perform research online by using search engines. If you don't get the results you were looking for, refine your search and try again.

Review Questions

1. What types of resources or activities would be helpful to someone who is an auditory learner?

2. What are at least three things you can do to make sure you're reading actively?

3. Which note-taking format would work best in a class where the instructor routinely gives a lot of anecdotes and examples to illustrate a single main idea?

4. How would you cope with an instructor who moved too slowly?

5. How does assessment software benefit students and instructors?

Chapter Activities

1. Discovering Your Learning Style: Login to the My Power Learning site (lww.mypowerlearning.com) and take the Learning Style Assessment. Print your Learning Style Index and specialized report.

2. Working Together: Divide into three groups based on your learning style assessment results (visual, auditory, or kinesthetic). In your group, come up with an idea for an activity or project that would help students with your learning style understand the information in this chapter. Then, write three to five sentences explaining how and why the activity or project would accommodate your particular learning style. Present your ideas to the other two groups in the class.

Chapter 5

ADVANCING THROUGH LISTENING, SPEAKING, WRITING, AND CRITICAL THINKING

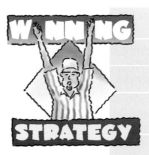

- Use active listening techniques in the classroom

- Adjust to different lecture styles

- Ask effective questions during class

- Discuss how participating in group discussions relates to speaking up in class

- Know why it's important for health care professionals to have good writing skills

- Create a schedule for completing a formal writing assignment

- Explain how critical thinking applies to a health care setting

- Describe Benjamin Bloom's six levels of cognitive learning

Listening, speaking, writing, and critical thinking skills are all necessary if you want to succeed as a student. During lectures, it may seem like your only responsibility is to sit quietly while your instructor speaks. This method might even have served you well in high school. But now you have the opportunity to do much more! By using the strategies discussed in this chapter, you'll be able to take charge of your own learning process. And when you're in control, nothing can stand in your way of learning new things and accomplishing your long-term goals. You'll be able to round the bases and slide safely into home!

Listening and Observation Survival Skills

To become an active participant in your own learning process, you'll need to do two things.

1. First, use strategies to help you listen actively in class. These strategies will help you take more effective notes and improve your level of listening.

2. Second, use your observation skills to help you adapt to difficult situations, such as dealing with a lecturer you find hard to follow.

By developing good listening and observation skills, you'll get more out of your courses.

STOP, LOOK, AND LISTEN

Active listening involves thinking about how you are listening and continually working to improve your listening skills. When you are listening actively in the classroom, you're doing more than simply hearing words. You're also deciphering main ideas, deciding which information is most important, and making adjustments in how you listen according to your instructor's teaching style.

In the game of school, an active listener is participating in the game, not just standing on the sidelines. Whether you need to become an active listener or merely improve your active listening skills, all students can follow these guidelines.

- Avoid doing things that can distract you from listening.
- Identify main ideas.
- Pay attention to the speaker's transition cues.
- Mentally organize information as you hear it and devote your attention to the material that seems more important.
- Take effective notes.

Interference!

There are several behaviors that could be sabotaging your active listening game. Make an effort to avoid:

- letting distractions interrupt your train of thought
- tuning out difficult material
- allowing your emotions to cloud your thinking
- automatically assuming the material is boring
- concentrating on the speaker's quirks
- letting your mind wander
- pretending to listen
- listening only for facts and not ideas
- trying to write down every word in your notes

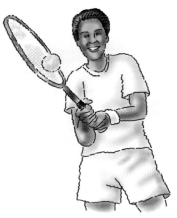

Avoid behaviors that could be hurting your active listening game. Keep your eye on the ball and stay focused!

Identify Main Ideas

Identifying main ideas is another element of active listening. Each lecture you hear will include main ideas even though they may be presented in different ways. Some of the approaches your instructor may take are:

- introducing new topics
- summarizing main points
- listing or discussing a main idea's supporting details
- showing two sides of the same issue
- discussing causes and effects related to a main idea
- identifying a main idea's problems and solutions

Wait for a Signal

Listening for signal words is another way to guide yourself through a lecture. These words are like play-by-play commentary in the classroom. They let you know which direction your instructor is headed.

Signal words can indicate transitions in a lecture. By paying attention to transitions, you'll be able to organize your thoughts and your notes as you listen actively. A few examples of signal words and phrases include:

- *Likewise*. This word indicates that the speaker is about to show how two concepts or examples are similar.
- *On the other hand*. If you hear this phrase or something similar to it, you'll know that the speaker is about to begin discussing an opposing fact or opinion.

- *Therefore*. This word usually indicates that the speaker is about to present an effect in a cause and effect relationship.
- *Finally*. This word lets you know that the speaker is arriving at the end of a point or the end of the lecture.

What Is Most Important?

Being able to separate more important information from less important information is a skill all active listeners need to possess. Instructors tend to have similar ways of communicating important information. Some write key terms and concepts on the chalkboard as they lecture. Other instructors distribute copies of lecture outlines at the beginning of class. By picking up on these clues, you'll have an easier time determining which information your instructor considers most important.

The following behaviors also can draw your attention to important material. Your instructor may:

- pause to allow students to copy information down in their notes
- repeat facts or definitions
- emphasize certain information with tone of voice
- directly tell students what information is important (for example, "Remember this for next Tuesday's test.")
- use gestures and facial expressions to draw attention to key information
- use visual aids, such as films, television segments, life-size plastic models, and information or images on projector screens
- have students turn to certain pages in the textbook

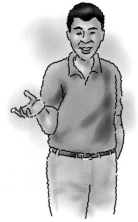

If your instructor repeats something, it's probably important information to remember.

Your instructor might not say, "This information is important." It's more likely that his behavior will give you the clues you'll need to figure out if it's important on your own. One way to pick up on these clues is to listen closely. Pay attention not only to your instructor's words, but to the tone and volume of his voice as well. Another way to notice clues about important material is to observe. Even if you are listening closely to every word your instructor says, if your head is buried in your notebook the whole time, you might miss certain clues. Instead, look up from your notes from time to time to observe your instructor's actions. Hand gestures and facial expressions can indicate important information almost as clearly as words.

LISAN and Learn

One of the benefits of active listening is that it will help you take more effective lecture notes. You learned about different note-taking methods in Chapter 4. When deciding how to format and take notes, make sure your note-taking method encourages active listening. The LISAN method of note-taking includes the following guidelines:

L   Lead instead of follow. Think about what your instructor might say next.

I   Ideas. What are the main ideas?

S   Signal words. Listen for signal words that indicate transitions in the lecture. In which direction is the lecture headed?

A   Actively listen. Make sure your mind stays engaged. Ask questions or make a note to yourself to seek clarification for difficult concepts later.

N   Notes. Write down main ideas, key terms, and any other important information. Be selective.

LISTENING LEVELS

Listening has to reach a certain level before it is considered active. Take a look at the chart below to see how well you listen in class. What level are you?

Level	Explanation
Reception	hearing words without thinking about them
Attention	passive listening; not making an effort to understand the information
Definition	entering into active listening; attaching meaning to certain facts and details but not yet organizing the material in your head
Integration	relating new information to your background knowledge
Interpretation	putting information into your own words; paraphrasing
Implication	thinking about how different pieces of information fit together; drawing conclusions
Application	considering how the information applies to you personally; using it in new situations
Evaluation	making judgments about the accuracy and relevance of the information

Remember that active listening is a learned skill. By following the tips in this chapter, you can learn to listen at a higher level. And once you know how to apply and evaluate information as you listen, you'll be that much further on your way to becoming a successful student!

LEARN TO ROLL WITH THE PUNCHES

In Chapter 4, you learned how to get the most out of your time in the classroom, regardless of the pace of each lecture or your instructor's speaking ability. This section discusses more tips for dealing with different lecturing styles.

During your time in school, you will come across many different types of instructors. One instructor may seem disorganized, whereas another doesn't cover the material in your textbook. Some instructors might not tell you exactly what you'll need to know for tests and quizzes. Although these situations may seem frustrating at first, you shouldn't use them as excuses to give up. To become a successful student, you'll need to learn to roll with the punches!

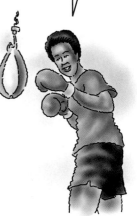

Jab, feint, weave, and watch your footwork! As a student, sometimes you have to roll with the punches.

When faced with these difficult situations, use them as opportunities to engage in your own learning process. When you're an active participant, you can achieve goals other than simply learning the required material. You can accomplish things such as:

- *Improving your learning skills.* You'll use these skills not only in school but in your future career as well. Remember, learning is a lifelong process!

- *Recognizing how lecture content is organized.* Whether your instructor follows the textbook, lectures independently of the text, or uses other media will determine what your learning focus should be in a particular class.

- *Discovering how to measure up to your instructor's expectations.* This also will be a useful skill to have once you become a practicing health care professional. In the future, you may not have to answer to an instructor, but you will want to know if you're meeting your supervisor's expectations.

Improve Your Learning Skills

Part of learning to roll with the punches involves improving your learning skills. Learning skills include:

- memorization
- the ability to apply new knowledge
- interpretation of difficult material
- the ability to identify different teaching styles

It may be that an instructor isn't necessarily an ineffective, or bad, lecturer, but one who presents material in a different way than your other instructors. Or, it may be that the material in a particular class requires a different style of teaching than you're used to. When this happens, look for clues to discover your instructor's teaching style. Then, use your different learning skills to help you adapt to the class.

Memorize It!

You'll probably find that a lot of memorization is required in your introductory courses. However, your instructors may not always specifically tell you which information to memorize. In these cases, look for clues to identify important information and commit it to memory.

For example, if your instructor writes a new concept or a definition on the chalkboard, you should make an effort to memorize it. Likewise, if your instructor distributes a handout depicting a diagram or a list of facts, it would be wise to remember that information as well. By learning early on to pay attention to your instructor's clues, you'll know exactly which material to memorize before the first quiz or test.

Apply It!

Some instructors focus on getting students to consider how the course material will apply to their future careers. If this is your instructor's goal, you'll do well in the course by showing that you can apply new knowledge. There are several ways in which your instructor might encourage you to do this.

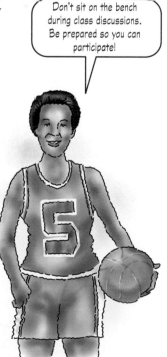

Don't sit on the bench during class discussions. Be prepared so you can participate!

- If your instructor gives many written assignments, be prepared to give examples of real-life applications in writing.

- If your instructor has students work through case studies during class, expect to see similar case studies on tests.

- If your instructor often calls students to the board to solve problems, be prepared to explain to the rest of the class how you would apply your new knowledge.

Interpret It!

In advanced science and health classes, instructors may ask students to interpret new information. This means you'll be expected to put ideas into your own words to show how well you understand the material. You'll recognize instructors who focus on interpretation by the fact that they often use class periods to ask questions and provide guidance on student responses. If your instructor uses this particular method, be sure to complete all assigned readings before class. Being prepared will allow you to participate in class discussions.

Know When to Shift Gears

Learning how to identify shifts in your instructor's teaching style will keep you alert and help you follow along with the lecture. For example, the notes you take during a class discussion will be different from the notes you take when your instructor gives you key terms and definitions to memorize. During a group discussion, you're focused more on ideas and the relationships between them. You won't be writing down every word that is said in class. In contrast, when your instructor gives you a definition to memorize, you'll need to either highlight the definition in your textbook or copy it word for word into your notes.

So, the next time your instructor interrupts a class discussion to write an important date or key term on the board, you'll know she's switching from an interpretive style of teaching to a memorization mode. You'll be able to adapt to this shift in teaching style by switching gears and recording the information from the board into your notes.

By listening actively, you'll soon become more familiar with your instructor's behavior. Pay attention to patterns in the way your instructor teaches. She may tell students directly that a particular concept is important. But she may give less obvious clues as well, such as becoming animated or using gestures while explaining important points. Once you can recognize shifts in your instructor's teaching style, you'll begin to get more out of each lecture.

Discover How Lecture Content Is Organized

The content in lectures can be organized in one of two ways:

1. *Text-dependent.* In lectures where the content is text-dependent, the material is presented very similarly to how it's presented in your textbook.

2. *Text-independent.* In these lectures, your instructor cites resources other than the text when presenting the information he considers most important.

Regardless of how closely their lectures follow the text, many instructors use media as well, to help them present lecture content.

A Textbook Case

If your instructor often conducts text-dependent lectures, it's especially important that you complete the assigned reading before class. If you're somewhat familiar with the material already, you'll have an easier time following along.

It's also important to bring your textbook to each class. As your instructor teaches, note important ideas in the margins of your text. You should highlight any passages or definitions your instructor reads aloud. If your instructor mentions that a particular section is unimportant or that you won't be required to know the information it contains, cross it out.

Some students don't like to mark up their books by writing in the margins or highlighting sections of text. This is because some college bookstores will buy back used textbooks at the end of the semester, and they'll only pay top dollar for books that haven't been marked in. At first, this may sound like a good plan for the budget-conscious student. However, carefully consider whether it's really worth it. Being able to highlight and quickly refer back to important lecture points may be well worth the few lost dollars. Also, by keeping your textbooks throughout your time at school, you'll find you have a terrific reference library to use later on in your professional career.

Beyond the Text

For lectures in which the content is text-independent, the focus shifts from your textbook to your notes. It's important to take effective notes during these lectures since you won't be able to refer back to your textbook for information you missed. After class, be sure to organize the lecture content by reviewing or outlining your notes. To gain a better understanding of the information, you may want to discuss each lecture with a class-mate—you could take turns "teaching" each other the material, which will help cement it in your brain. You also could use supplementary material, such as computer software or online articles, to review concepts presented by your instructor. (See *Using Supplemental Material* in Chapter 4.)

Before you sit down to study the material, set a few study goals to remind yourself what pieces of information you need to learn. This is essential when dealing with content that doesn't appear in your textbook. You'll need to create your own learning objectives for the information in your lecture notes, as the chapter objectives from your textbook may not apply.

A Media Frenzy

A third element that affects lecture content is the use of media. Handouts, films, slide or PowerPoint presentations, plastic models, and other forms of media give students new ways of learning about the material. For example, a movie might cause you to have an emotional response to a certain topic while a plastic model might give you an opportunity to practice your clinical skills. With each form of media, you're able to connect to the material in a different way. Often, this allows you to learn and understand more information than you would by simply hearing your instructor discuss it.

When dealing with media in the classroom, there are two things on which you should focus. Ask yourself:

- Why is the instructor using this particular medium?
- How does this medium meet my learning needs?

For instance, suppose your instructor plays a television segment during class. If the segment is about a topic you've already covered, it can help you review necessary information. But if the segment introduces a new topic, it can meet your learning needs by providing you with background knowledge.

Find Out How to Measure Up

It's a good idea to set up a conference with your instructor at least once during the semester or term. A student-teacher conference gives you the opportunity to ask questions about lecture content, learn about your instructor's expectations of students, or discuss any other important issues related to the course.

Here are a few tips to consider when scheduling a conference.

- Decide on a specific topic to discuss, such as your first test or a confusing concept from a recent lecture.
- Write down any questions you'd like to ask about that topic, putting your most important questions at the top of the list. Your instructor may have a limited amount of time to meet with you.

Schedule a student-teacher conference to learn more about what your instructor expects of students.

If you're organized and prepared for the meeting, you'll have a better chance of getting the information you need in that short period of time. Also, if the idea of a student-teacher conference makes you nervous, having questions already written out will put your mind at ease and help you stay focused.

By taking initiative and meeting with your instructor one on one, you'll demonstrate that you're concerned about your success as a student. You'll also gain a better understanding of your instructor. This will help you make sure you're

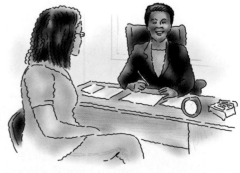

on the same wavelength—it's always better to be aware of your instructor's expectations than to blindly assume you're doing well in a course.

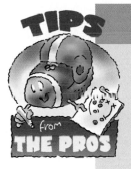

TAKING UP THE SLACK

If a speaker is hard to follow, pick up the slack in the lecture by using the strategies listed below.

If your instructor doesn't...	You should...
explain goals for the day's lecture	set goals yourself by referring to your textbook or syllabus
go over information covered in the previous lecture	review your lecture notes for a few minutes before each class
provide an introduction or summary at the beginning and end of a lecture	write a brief summary of each lecture after class
supply students with an outline of each lecture	review the assigned reading before class or outline your notes after the day's lecture
give students enough time to write notes before moving on to the next topic	speak up!; politely ask your instructor to repeat or clarify information
speak in a clear, loud tone of voice	politely ask your instructor to speak louder, or move to a closer seat, as long as you don't disrupt the class
answer students' questions without being sarcastic or discouraging	avoid taking your instructor's remarks personally
stay on topic and instead begins talking about personal experiences	think about how the instructor's stories relate to the topic
explain the chapter and instead reads directly from the textbook	follow along by highlighting the text your instructor reads; outline or summarize the text in your notes
provide the main points of the lecture	reread your textbook after class and locate main points
clarify confusing information or provide examples	ask your instructor to provide an example or come up with an example on your own
write key terms and definitions on the chalkboard	look up key terms in a dictionary or in the glossary of your textbook

The Essentials of Expressing Yourself

To succeed as a student, you'll need to learn how to express yourself through speaking and writing.

SPEAKING

During your time as a student, you may be required to give a few speeches or oral presentations. However, most of the public speaking you do will be on a more informal level. Whether you're asking a question during a lecture or participating in a group discussion, you should use good public speaking skills. By being able to express yourself, you'll obtain sufficient answers to your questions and you'll also get more out of group discussions.

Me? Speak in Public?

If speaking to a group of people makes you feel nervous, nauseous, or as if you'd rather stay in bed and avoid the situation altogether, know that you're not alone. *Glossophobia*, or the fear of public speaking, is considered by some to be the most common phobia.

Researchers aren't sure exactly what causes this fear. However, most agree that having a bad or embarrassing experience with public speaking is usually a major contributor. There's nothing like the embarrassment of getting up in front of a group of people and stumbling over your words (or forgetting them altogether) to make you want to avoid doing so ever again.

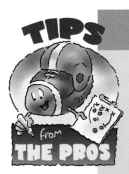

LEARNING TO SPEAK UP

Follow this step-by-step process to relax yourself before speaking up in class.

- Acknowledge your fears and admit to yourself that you're nervous. It's very difficult to overcome a fear that "doesn't exist."

- Reassure yourself that you have something important to say and that your instructor and your classmates are interested in hearing it.

- Think about what you are going to say. This will give you a chance to calm your nerves.

- Be confident. This will command everyone's interest.

- Speak loudly and clearly. If everyone hears you the first time, you will avoid having to repeat yourself.

Fortunately, there are tips you can use to improve your ability to speak up in a group setting.

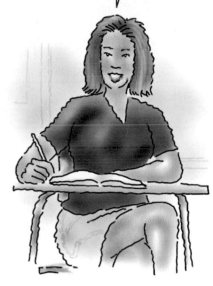

Before speaking up in class, take a moment to organize your thoughts.

Organize Your Thoughts

The first thing to remember is to organize your thoughts. During lectures, pay attention and listen closely to make sure your instructor hasn't already addressed the question you're about to ask. Then, ask directly. There is no need to beat around the bush. Go ahead and ask for clarification of an idea or challenge a statement that seems contradictory. In most classrooms, it's acceptable and even encouraged for students to participate in this way.

Come to the Point

As you learned in Chapter 4, there's a right way and a wrong way to go about seeking clarification during a lecture. The wrong way would be to interrupt class with a vague statement such as, "I don't get it." Here's the best way to ask a question.

1. State briefly and in your own words the part of the material you *do* understand.
2. Then, come to the point by asking a specific question.

For example, suppose your radiology instructor is explaining how to position patients for different types of x-rays. If you need clarification, you could say, "I understand that in both the recumbent and supine positions, the patient should be lying down. But what is the difference between the two positions?" This statement clearly shows that you understand at least part of the information. It's an effective question because it comes to the point and tells your instructor exactly which part of the material you don't understand.

On the other hand, suppose you encounter a situation where you want to challenge a statement that seems to contradict your background knowledge of a particular topic. Let's say your class is having a discussion about patient privacy rights. Your instructor says, "State law requires that if a patient is diagnosed with a sexually transmitted disease, that information must be reported to the local health department." In a previous course, however, you learned that a patient's diagnosis is confidential. Your instructor's statement seems to contradict what you've already learned about patient confidentiality. How would you form a respectful question to challenge your instructor's statement?

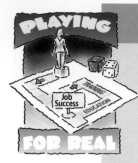

SPEAKING UP

Hi, my name is Suki. I'm studying to become a lab technician. In one of the first courses I took, it was really hard to keep up with the instructor. But I was afraid to ask questions in front of everyone else in class. The few times I tried, I was so nervous that I raised my hand and then completely forgot what I was going to say.

But then I started writing down my questions so I could read them after the instructor called on me. It was so much easier! Writing down what I wanted to say gave me the time I needed to organize my thoughts. It also kept me from being too nervous and having my mind go blank.

Participate—Group Discussions

A good way to practice speaking up in class is to participate in group discussions with your classmates. These situations provide you with lower stress opportunities to express your thoughts and ask questions. Once you become comfortable with speaking to a group of your peers, you'll gain confidence to speak up in other situations, such as asking your instructor for clarification.

For Future Use

The speaking skills you develop as a student will be useful throughout your career. When the situation arises where you need to clarify a physician's instructions, you'll be thankful for all the practice you had in class communicating with your instructors! As a health care professional, you'll need to apply the same principles you used in class when asking your supervisors for clarification.

1. First, organize your thoughts in order to ask a direct question.

2. Then, come to the point while remembering to be respectful and to use your critical thinking skills.

You'll also need to have good speaking skills to help you communicate with patients. For example, when gathering a patient's medical history, you'll be required to ask direct questions and clarify the patient's responses. In this case, you'll need to be able to form clear, easily understandable questions to obtain the information you need. It also will be important to make sure you understand the patient's responses correctly before recording the information in a medical chart.

Good speaking skills, and good communication skills in general, are very important in health care professions. Eventually, you'll be required to use your skills on a daily basis. Just remember that the best way to develop good skills is to practice!

WRITING

As a student, you'll most likely be required to write essays, reports, and research papers. The writing skills you develop in school can be carried into your professional career as well. As a health professional, you'll need to have solid writing skills for the purpose of recording accurate and concise information in patient charts and medical records.

Writing skills can be helpful for a number of other reasons, one of which is securing your first job. A well-written resume and cover letter can help you get your foot in the door and get an interview. Another practical application of your writing skills would be sending e-mail messages. Being able to express yourself well through your writing shows that you are intelligent and competent. It also effectively gets your message across to the person with whom you are communicating. Good writing skills help you avoid the misunderstandings that can result from poor communication.

Structurally Speaking

Whether you're writing a 15-page paper or a brief essay, your writing assignments should be structured in roughly the same way. Formal writing includes an introduction, a body, and a conclusion.

Introduction

Make sure your formal written assignments always begin with an introduction. The introduction should interest the reader in the topic you're about to discuss. Your introduction can be structured in a number of different ways. It can:

- be centered on a thesis statement (a thesis statement is a statement of the opinion or idea to be discussed in your paper)
- present a problem or ask a question that you intend to answer
- describe a dramatic event or incident
- provide interesting statistics
- set a scene
- relate a short story

For example, in a persuasive essay, your introduction could begin by presenting a topic. Then, your thesis statement could include the main point you intend to prove about that topic.

One important thing to keep in mind about your introduction is that it doesn't have to be the first thing you write. Even if you start with a basic outline and have a general idea of how you'd like to approach your topic, it's easy to get stuck on the introduction. If this happens, try working on other portions of the paper for a while and come back to it. Your introduction will be easier to write once you have a clear purpose in mind.

In terms of length, the introduction should be roughly 5 to 15 percent of the length of your entire paper. It needs to be informative, but to the point. It should be interesting without giving away too much detail. Because of these reasons, it takes time and effort to write a good introduction. You may want to look over it again and make any necessary revisions after you've completed your paper.

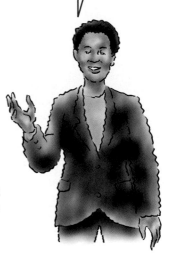

Spice up your introduction by beginning with a brief story, asking a question, or presenting an interesting fact.

Body

You will do most of your writing in the body. This part makes up about 70 to 90% of a paper's total length. The body of a paper presents details that support your thesis. These details may include:

- background information about your topic
- facts and supporting research
- explanations of key terms or phrases used throughout the paper
- quotes from other credible sources
- different arguments against your thesis and your responses to those arguments

Conclusion

A strong conclusion ends the discussion presented in the paper and makes the reader think. To accomplish this, the conclusion needs to do more than blandly summarize main points. To write a strong conclusion, consider including:

- a quotation that relates to or sums up your thesis
- a question for the reader to consider
- encouragement for the reader to act in support of your idea
- one last example or story to reiterate your point

Bibliography

The bibliography is a list of the sources you used to write your paper. It's important because it helps you back up the information included in your paper and gives credit to the people whose research or quotes you cited. Whether you gathered information from a book, a Web site, a television program, or a magazine article, each source must be included in your bibliography.

Appendix

You probably won't need to include an appendix with each formal writing assignment you complete. An appendix is only necessary when you need to include other supportive materials that do not belong, or cannot fit, in the body of your paper. A few examples of such materials are:

- a list of key terms and definitions
- photos, illustrations, or figures
- tables, charts, maps, and other graphic elements

The Writing Process

So you've decided on the type of paper you're going to write. You know it needs to have an introduction, a body, and a conclusion. What next? There are several steps to follow in the process of writing a paper.

1. Determine a schedule.
2. Select a topic.
3. Collect information.
4. Organize the information.
5. Evaluate the information.
6. Create an outline.
7. Write a first draft.
8. Revise the first draft.
9. Finalize the paper.

Scheduling

A good way to set up a schedule for writing a paper is to work backwards. First, look up the due date for the paper in your syllabus. Then, mark the following on your school calendar:

- due date for the paper
- amount of time you need to revise the paper
- amount of time you need to write the first draft

- date you should complete your research
- date you need to begin research

When scheduling your time, be generous! Unexpected problems can arise, making certain steps take longer than you anticipated. For example, you may go to the library to find that a book you need has already been checked out. Or you may find that you need extra time to evaluate and organize the materials you gathered. Whatever the case may be, you can avoid stress by allowing yourself enough time to plan for delays during the writing process.

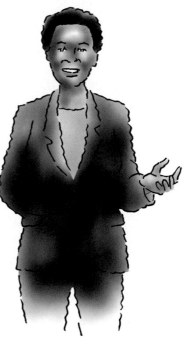

Use the required page length to help you figure out how long it will take you to write the paper.

Another aspect that may affect your writing schedule is the paper's length. Sometimes it's hard to predict how much work you'll need to do to complete the assignment. When considering how much time to allow yourself to write the paper, keep the following in mind:

- the required length of the paper
- the amount of time you have before the due date
- the amount of research you're expected to do
- the number of references your instructor requires you to have

Selecting a Topic

If your instructor assigns a specific topic, you won't have to worry about this stage of the writing process. If not, your instructor may provide you with a list of acceptable topics or with guidelines for creating your own topic. When thinking about possible topics for your paper, select one that captures your interest. By writing about a subject that interests you, you'll be better motivated to work on the paper. Also, be sure to select a topic that you'll be able to research adequately. You'll have a hard time completing an assignment that requires a lot of research if your topic is very obscure.

Good places to search for topic ideas include:

- the table of contents in your textbook
- your lecture notes
- brainstorming sessions with your study group
- magazines, newspapers, or television

Just remember to keep your topic fairly narrow. A more focused topic means a more focused writing process and a better paper. When looking for a topic, try to find a balance. Your topic should provide you with enough material to complete the assignment but it should be focused enough so that you can explain it fully in your paper.

One way to see if a topic is well defined or focused enough is to think about your thesis statement and the title of the paper. A good title should be clear and appealing. The reader should know what the paper is about just by reading the title. However, if you come up with a title before writing the paper, keep in mind that the title isn't permanent. You can always change the title after the paper has been completed. Sometimes, it's simply a good exercise to think about the main point you'd like to communicate in your paper. Doing so may help you decide on a particular topic.

Collecting Information

When gathering information for your paper, it's probably wise to begin at the library. Start by looking up your topic in the library's computer system. Another good reference is the *Reader's Guide to Periodical Literature*. This book lists the titles and subjects of magazine and journal articles. Your library also should have a set of encyclopedias and some specialized dictionaries in its reference section.

If you have trouble locating these resources at the library, the reference librarian is there to help. He can offer you research tips as well as educate you on how to use the library.

OTHER SOURCES OF INFORMATION

Aside from the library, other excellent sources of information are:

- *Interviews with professors or experts in the field.* Conducting interviews will prepare you for future clinical work, when you may have to conduct information-gathering interviews with patients. In both cases, the process is similar.
  1. First, be prepared. Make a list of the questions you'd like to ask. Make sure the most important questions are at the top of your list.
  2. During the interview, keep the conversation focused. If you only have a limited amount of time, try to avoid talking about things unrelated to your questions.
  3. Finally, when gathering information for a paper, you may wish to audiotape the interview in addition to taking notes. This can help you remember quotes accu-

rately. It also gives you a way to review any information you may have missed. Just remember to ask permission first. You can do this when scheduling the interview to avoid putting your interviewee on the spot when you meet; not everyone is comfortable with being recorded.

- *Surveys and statistics.* You can use the results of professional surveys when collecting information for your paper. But you can conduct your own surveys as well. Statistics can be calculated after you receive responses to your survey. For example, suppose you surveyed 50 subjects and 15 of those individuals answered *yes* to a particular question. The other 35 subjects answered *no.* Your statistics for that question would be 30 percent ($15 \div 50 = .30$) of subjects answered *yes* and 70 percent ($35 \div 50 = .70$) answered *no.* These results could then be used in your paper to prove or disprove a particular point.

- *Resources on the Internet.* When searching for information online, there are two very important guidelines to keep in mind.
  1. First, make sure the material you find is reliable. (See the *Web Sites* section in Chapter 4.)
  2. Second, remember to cite any online information you use in your paper. Your instructor will be able to tell you which format to use when citing information. You'll most likely need to include the Web address, site owner, date the site was last updated (if available), and the date you accessed the information.

- *Unbiased observations.* Your unbiased observations can be used as a source of information for your paper. However, the key word here is *unbiased.* There are several methods you can use to avoid allowing your own opinions to cloud your observations. For example, you could create a checklist of things to look for as you observe a certain situation. During your observation, use the checklist to guide your note-taking. Having a checklist and thorough notes will add reliability to your observations.

- *Personal experiences.* Some instructors will allow you to use information gathered from your own experiences. Just be sure the experiences you draw from are directly related to the topic of your paper. Also, back up your experiences with more objective information from sources you trust, such as reference books or articles in academic journals.

Organizing Your Information

To begin organizing your information, use index cards. Fill out one index card per source, including main ideas and references to page numbers. (You'll need to know page numbers when creating your bibliography or citing sources within your paper.)

Start by creating cards for your general sources and then move to more specific sources. This is a good time to take notes on each source and look for quotes as well. Be sure to copy down quotes word for word and cite them accurately on your index cards. In the sources themselves, use sticky notes to mark relevant chapters or sections. For photocopied pages, you can use colorful highlighters to mark important information.

Next, organize your index cards according to topic. If you have several sources that provide the same information, discard the ones you won't need. Also, begin thinking about the basic layout of your paper at this point. Separate your cards into three stacks.

- The first stack will be for information that belongs toward the beginning of your paper.
- The second stack will be for material you plan to use toward the middle of your paper.
- The third stack will hold the cards you'll need to consult when writing the end of your paper.

> Try using a color-coding system or symbols to keep your index cards organized. Just be creative and use a method that works easily for you.

Evaluating Your Information

After you've organized your sources, you'll need to check each one for relevance to your topic. This includes:

- checking the publication date (if possible, try to avoid using sources published more than 5 years ago)
- making sure each source contains supporting information

If you find a source that argues against your thesis, it may still be relevant to your paper. You can write a stronger paper by including differing points of view and defending your thesis. Sources that contain counterpoint material also help you determine how well your thesis holds up against arguments. If you find that your thesis is too weak, this is a good point in the writing process to rethink the focus of your paper. It would be much easier to rewrite your thesis than it would be to try and write an entire paper about an idea you're unable to support.

Once you've separated out the relevant sources, make sure the information they contain is reliable. As you review each source, ask yourself:

- *Is the author biased?* Does the author merely present her personal opinions without backing up her statements with facts or research? Does the author criticize certain ideas without giving solid reasons why those ideas are faulty? Have statistics been presented in a misleading way to further the author's opinion?

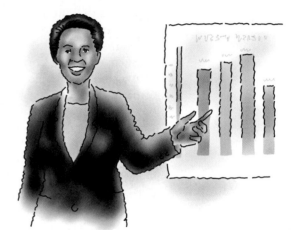

Remember that statistics can be manipulated. Even if information is presented as fact, you still need to evaluate it!

- *Is the source primary or secondary?* A primary source contains first-hand information. A secondary source restates material from a primary source. Occasionally, secondary sources reproduce quotes made in primary sources. Out of context, those quotes may take on different meanings, which affect their reliability. Whenever possible, use primary sources.

After evaluating your sources, keep only those that contain reliable information important to your topic. Then, set aside those index cards for sources you've decided not to use. Later, when you're sure you're not going to need those sources, you can discard them.

Creating an Outline

The next stage in the writing process is creating an outline. Your thesis statement can serve as the outline's introduction. This will help you stay focused on your main point as you write the rest of the outline. Another way to keep your writing focused is to write a brief conclusion. You can expand this conclusion later when you write the first draft of your paper.

Next, refer to your index card notes as you map out the body of the outline. If you're required to submit a title page, table of contents, appendix, or bibliography with your final paper, use simple one-line entries to note these items on your outline as well.

When deciding how to organize the body of your outline, think about your three different stacks of index cards.

- The cards in the first stack will provide you with material for the beginning of your paper.
- The cards in the second stack will be used for writing the middle.
- The cards in the third stack will provide information for the end.

As you write your outline, and even as you write your paper, you're free to move sections around and reorganize information. The purpose of having an outline is to give yourself a guide. But it isn't set in stone. An outline allows you to see the organization of your paper at a glance and make necessary changes before you begin writing your first draft.

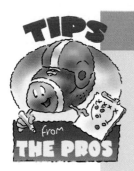

ANATOMY OF AN OUTLINE

Follow these tips when creating an outline for your paper.

I. Creating an outline
   A. Sections
      1. Introduction (use thesis statement)
      2. Body (consult index cards)
      3. Conclusion
      4. Other items (one-line entries)
         a. title page
         b. table of contents
         c. appendix
         d. bibliography
   B. Organization
      1. Use index cards to organize info in the body
         a. beginning of paper (first stack of cards)
         b. middle of paper (second stack of cards)
         c. end of paper (third stack of cards)
      2. Move sections around as necessary

Writing a First Draft

The first draft of your paper is just that—a draft. Don't worry about editing and polishing your writing at this point. There will be plenty of time for that later. The most important thing is to begin putting your ideas into sentences and paragraphs.

While writing the first draft, you'll develop the introduction and body of your paper. You'll need to begin keeping track of footnotes (if they are required by your instructor) and bibliographic references. You'll also expand on the brief conclusion you wrote for your outline.

Another important part of writing a first draft involves developing the tone you'll use throughout your paper. To do this, think about your audience. Is this paper intended for your instructor? Will you be presenting it to the rest of the class? To have a consistent tone in all sections of your paper, keep your audience in mind as you write.

Your outline will guide the process of writing a first draft. As you begin writing, however, feel free to make changes if the organization of your outline isn't working. If you use a computer to type your first draft, it will be easy to move sections of text. Just remember to save your work often! It's also a good idea to back up your writing on disk or by some other method.

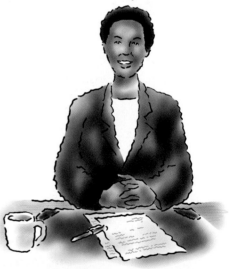

The wheels in your head will keep turning even after you take a break from your paper. After you finish the first draft, put it away for a while and let your brain keep working.

The last step in writing your first draft is to put it away for a while. Depending on your schedule, this may mean 24 hours or several days. This gives your brain time to process what you've written. During the time you spend away from writing, you may think of ways to improve your paper. Whether you come up with the perfect introduction or a better way to state your conclusion, these ideas are valuable. Write them down so you can incorporate them later as you make revisions to your first draft.

Revising the First Draft

After you've given yourself some time away from your paper, you can begin writing the second draft. By this time, you should have a better idea of how the overall organization of your paper is working. If any big organizational changes need to be made, now is the time to make them.

Again, if you're working on a computer, remember to save often! Another helpful tip for computer users is to rename each draft (for example, Draft 1, Draft 2, Draft 3, etc.). That way, you'll always be able to refer to a previous version of your paper if you delete a section by mistake or if you decide to go back to your original organization plan.

With each draft, your paper should resemble more closely how it will look in its final stage. But how many drafts is enough? Reading your entire paper aloud is one way to help you notice parts that may need improvement. As you read, look at the following qualities:

- *Organization*. Does the overall organization make sense? Does the paper move forward in a logical and clear way?

- *Paragraph structure*. Does each paragraph have a main idea and supporting details? Does the paper include transitions from one paragraph to the next?

- *Sentence flow*. Do the sentences flow smoothly from one to the next?

As you consider how many times to revise your paper, also keep the due date in mind. Be sure to allow yourself enough time for editing.

Once you're satisfied with the body of your paper, it's time to create the title page, table of contents (page numbers can be inserted after your final edit), bibliography, appendix, and any other items required by your instructor. Then, have someone else read the paper—it's always a good idea to have a fresh pair of eyes look for anything you may have missed. Your reviewer can look at things, such as spelling, grammar, organization, logic, and any other elements your instructor may use to grade the paper. But keep in mind that any suggestions made by your reviewer are merely suggestions. In the end, you decide which changes to make to your paper.

> Well, I'm satisfied with this paper. Now I just need someone else to review it.

Finalizing the Paper

The final stage in the writing process involves editing, formatting, and proofreading your paper.

1. During editing, it's helpful to consult other resources, such as a dictionary, thesaurus, and an English grammar and usage guide. These resources should be available in the reference section of the library. As you edit your work, follow these guidelines.

   - Check the paper's tone to make sure it remains consistent.

   - Make sure terms are used consistently throughout the paper. For example, if you used *congestive heart failure* in one paragraph, avoid changing it to *heart failure* in another paragraph if it refers to the same condition.

- Spell check your paper. Check any words the spell checker doesn't recognize (such as scientific terms).
- Check your grammar. Make sure all singular subjects have singular verbs and all plural subjects have plural verbs.
- Check your punctuation. All sentences should end with a period or other punctuation mark. All text in quotes should have both opening and closing quotation marks.
- Check the spacing between lines of text. Most instructors require students to use double spacing to allow plenty of room for marks and comments.
- Make sure the font size is appropriate (12 pt. font is standard).

2. The next step in finalizing your paper is formatting. Use the following tips as you format your paper.

- Follow your instructor's formatting guidelines. If specific guidelines aren't provided, your instructor may require you to adhere to a particular style manual instead (such as the *Publication Manual of the American Psychological Association*). Style manuals can answer questions you may have about specialized terms and industry style and formatting standards. These resources also can be found in the reference section of the library.
- Print a hard copy of your paper. Reviewing a hard copy will be easier on your eyes than looking at your paper on a computer screen. Additionally, formatting errors become much more visible in a printed copy.

3. Take a short break before you begin the last step—proofreading. If you're too familiar with the text of your paper, your eyes might begin to skip over errors. By allowing yourself a break, you'll come back refreshed and ready to read your paper closely. Here are some proofreading tips.

- Read your entire paper aloud (if possible).
- Be on the lookout for any errors in punctuation or capitalization.
- When you come across an unfamiliar word, look it up in the dictionary to check its spelling and meaning.

After this last step has been completed, you can hand in your final paper feeling confident about your work!

Participate—Group Projects

When group writing projects are assigned, your main focus should be on acting as a dependable teammate. Not only will you need to contribute quality written material, you'll need to offer your input to the rest of the group and complete your work on time.

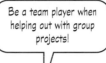

Be a team player when helping out with group projects!

As you learned in Chapter 2, study group members need to be *committed contributors* who are *compatible* with one another and *considerate* of each other. The same is true when working with a group of your class-mates on a writing assignment.

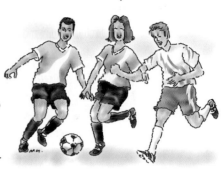

1. First and foremost, everyone in the group needs to be committed to the project.

2. Second, each person is responsible for bringing something to the table by sup-plying ideas and written material.

3. Third, even if your instructor assigned you to work with a group of people you don't get along with, you should find a way to overlook your differences and focus on the project.

4. Finally, if everyone in the group makes an effort to speak politely and be considerate of each other's time, the proj-ect will go smoothly.

Critical Thinking—Why Is It So Important?

It's especially important for health care professionals to have solid critical thinking skills. When you think critically, you ana-lyze information to form judgments about it. The information may be gathered from your observations, personal experience, reasoning, or communication. In your profession, you may be required to gather and analyze information and evaluate results on a daily basis. If you're able to think critically and make good judgments based on the information you can gather, you'll have a positive impact on your patients' health.

DIRECT YOURSELF TO LEARNING

Individuals who are successful in both school and the work-place have achieved their success by becoming self-directed

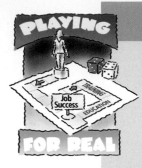

CRITICAL THINKING SKILLS IN THE WORKPLACE

My name is Derek. I've been working as a certified medical assistant for about a year now, and I've definitely had to put my critical thinking skills to the test! I work in a family practice office, so our patients are all ages and they come in for a lot of different reasons.

Last week, one of our patients made an appointment because he was experiencing abdominal pain. He arrived early for his appointment, and said he was still experiencing pain and that he was feeling nauseous, too. I could tell he was in obvious distress—his skin was pale and he was holding his stomach in pain. Even though his appointment time wasn't for another 20 minutes, I decided to take him back to wait in an empty exam room. Then, I gave the physician a heads-up about his symptoms, in case he needed to be examined right away. It's a good thing I did, because as it turned out, the patient had appendicitis!

learners. Being a self-directed learner means that you take responsibility for your own education. You've already read about several ways to accomplish this.

For example, if you're having a hard time understanding a particular concept in class, you can find other resources, ask your instructor for clarification, or meet with your study group. Although test scores are important, your main goal in school should be to learn the material. Being a self-directed learner means not only studying in order to do well on tests and quizzes, but also studying in order to store information in your long-term memory. It also means being able to apply that information to new situations once you become a practicing health care professional.

Likewise, successful professionals must be self-directed learners. Once you are no longer a student, you'll have to take even more responsibility for your own learning. This may mean keeping yourself up-to-date on the latest research by reading articles related to your field. Or it may mean requesting to observe a procedure you've been struggling to learn. In these cases, you should be aware of what you need to learn and how you can go about increasing your knowledge and improving your skills.

Regardless of your past experience as a student, you can achieve success now by becoming a self-directed learner. You have clearly chosen to be here today because of your motivation toward a particular career goal. Contrary to how you may feel at first, you *can* control a great deal of what you learn and how your educational experience will unfold.

Learning is a process. By understanding how the process works, you can begin to develop the learning skills you'll use as a student and later in your professional career.

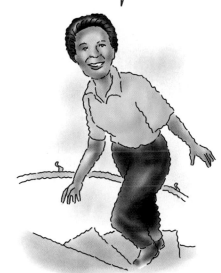

Learning is a process. You have to start at the bottom and work your way up to the next level.

BLOOM'S LEARNING LEVELS

Cognitive learning, or critical thinking, occurs in several stages. Benjamin Bloom, a noted neuropsychologist, assigned names and descriptions to these stages in the 1950s.

- knowledge
- comprehension
- application
- analysis
- synthesis
- evaluation

Although other psychologists have developed new theories about critical thinking since the 1950s, most theories are similar to Bloom's. In other theories, the stages may be named or ordered differently, but their descriptions remain relatively the same.

Knowledge

During the knowledge stage of critical thinking, you memorize information and repeat it word for word. At this point, you don't necessarily have to understand the information to memorize it. Some examples of things you may need to memorize are:

- formulas in a math class
- people's names, addresses, and phone numbers
- simple instructions

Comprehension

In the comprehension stage of critical thinking, you're able to understand information enough to restate it in your own words. If you take effective notes during class, your notes should reflect your comprehension. You can accomplish this by:

- drawing charts and diagrams
- summarizing and paraphrasing information
- describing how concepts are related
- explaining the material to someone else

Application

During this stage, you use the information you've memorized and comprehended to accomplish a task. Examples of application include:

- using a mathematic formula to solve a problem
- using a rule or principle to classify information
- successfully completing a project by following directions

Analysis

Analysis involves taking information and breaking it into parts to understand how those parts are organized and related to one another. For example, when you read an article in a magazine, you first look at the different pieces of information presented. An author may provide several anecdotes to illustrate a single main point. Then, you analyze the different pieces of information by thinking about how they are related. How does each anecdote relate to the author's theme or main point? What message is the author trying to get across?

Synthesis

In the synthesis stage of critical thinking, you put your analysis to use by developing a new idea. In a sense, you take parts of information and put them together in a different way to form a new concept. This stage of learning is more creative than the others. It includes:

- building on the pieces of information contained in your notes and writing a paper or presentation
- forming a plan for conducting a lab experiment
- writing a poem or short story

Evaluation

During the last stage in the critical thinking process, you evaluate information. This means you use other methods, such as comprehension and analysis, to determine whether or not information has value or relevance. Evaluation can include:

- determining which conclusions are actually supported by facts and research

- judging the value of a work of art or a piece of writing based on specific standards
- determining the value and relevance of information presented in a textbook, lecture, or class discussion

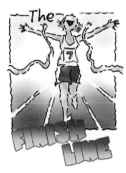

- Avoid behaviors that can interfere with active listening.
- When listening actively, identify main ideas and pay attention to signal words.
- Make appropriate adjustments when you notice shifts in your instructor's teaching style.
- Schedule student-teacher conferences to ask your instructor for clarification, discuss your academic performance in a course, or learn more about your instructor's expectations of students.
- Use techniques to compensate for different lecture styles and become an active participant in your own learning process.
- Improve your ability to express yourself by speaking up during class and participating in group discussions with your peers.
- Develop good writing skills now for later use in a health care setting, such as writing accurate and concise reports in patient charts.
- Create detailed schedules to help you complete formal writing assignments properly and meet deadlines set by your instructor.
- Be a dependable team player when group writing projects are assigned. Participate by giving your input, completing your work on time, and being sure to contribute quality written material.
- Use critical thinking to assess and judge information before making a decision about the facts. By improving your critical thinking skills now, you'll have a positive effect on your patients' health once you become a health care professional.
- Become a self-directed learner by taking control of your education and reaching for your goals.

Remember, critical thinking is a tool used not just by students, but by health care professionals as well.

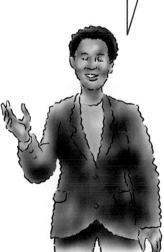

Review Questions

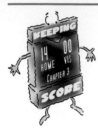

1. What are at least five behaviors that could be interfering with your ability to listen actively in class?

2. When gathering material for a paper, what are several sources of information you can use aside from the library?

3. Write a definition for critical thinking in your own words.

Chapter Activities

1. Critical Thinking Exercise: Review *Bloom's Learning Levels*. Draw a pyramid, set of stairs, skyscraper, or another image to illustrate Bloom's six levels of learning. Then, label each level and provide a practical example. For instance, a practical example for the lowest level of learning, knowledge, could be memorizing the definition of a key term and repeating it word for word.

2. Group Discussion: Begin with a warm-up exercise to get everyone participating. Think of something, aside from family and friends, that you value (such as a painting, CD collection, book, etc.). Then, in 1 to 2 minutes, share with the rest of the class what that object is and why it's important to you. After everyone has had a chance to participate in the warm-up exercise, discuss as a group several reasons why people may have a fear of public speaking. Why is the ability to speak up particularly important in a health care setting?

Chapter 6

STRATEGIC STUDYING

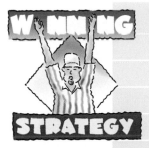

- Select and prepare a study space

- Improve your concentration

- Learn ways to improve your memorization skills

- Explore different study strategies

- Improve your efficiency as you study

- Grasp how, when, and where to network

- Take advantage of free study resources

Much of your time as a student will be spent studying. If the thought of studying makes you groan, don't despair! There are many simple strategies you can use to make the most of your study time and the resources available to you. In this chapter, you'll learn how to get started: how to select a study space and how to prepare yourself to begin studying. You'll learn tips for improving your concentration and long-term memory as well.

This chapter also explains how to create a network that can benefit your studies while helping you share what you've learned with others. People in your network can be great resources of information, advice, and support. Other resources covered in this chapter include your instructor's office hours and special services offered by your school, along with Internet resources and text-book software. As you'll learn in this chapter, the key to making use of the resources available to you is knowing where to look and then taking the initiative to seek them out.

Studying 101

Studying seems simple: get out your books and notes and study them. But what does it really mean to study? Studying is:

- refreshing your memory
- taking in new information
- organizing and memorizing data

That's a lot! It's no surprise that many students sit down to study and find themselves feeling overwhelmed. Any little distraction can throw a wrench in the works, keeping students from studying efficiently. That's why it's important to study the right way.

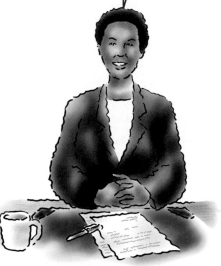

When it comes to studying, think, *location, location, location!* Finding a good place to study is just as important as the study methods you use.

SCOPE OUT A STUDY AREA

The first thing you need to do is find a good place to study. Look for a location that is free of distractions. (See *How to Find a Distraction-Free Study Zone.*) Also, make sure the area is large enough for you to arrange all your study materials. Think about any furniture you might need, such as a desk or large table.

For example, some students prefer to sit at a table when they study. This arrangement keeps them alert and focused, while helping them keep their materials organized. They can put the study materials they're using on the table and keep materials they'll need later underneath it. Other students, however, might feel more comfortable sitting on a sofa, with their study materials on a coffee table or spread out on the floor below. One place you may want to avoid studying, if you can, is your bedroom. If you're tired, your bed will be calling you to take a nap!

After you've come up with several possible study areas, compare each space in terms of the lighting, temperature, and other surroundings.

Lighting

Make sure your study space has good lighting you can control. Light is very important. Too much will make your eyes hurt, while too little will make your eyes strain. The light should shine evenly over all your work and not directly into your eyes.

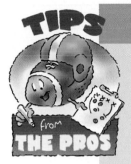

HOW TO FIND A DISTRACTION-FREE STUDY ZONE

Think about two or three areas that might make good study spaces. Then choose the one place that has the most favorable responses to these questions.

- Are there a lot of other people in the same space who could interrupt me?
- Are there things in the space that will distract me from studying?
- Is there a TV or radio in the space that might be turned on?
- Is there a phone that might ring too often?
- Is this space easy for me to get to on a regular basis?
- Is the temperature comfortable? If it isn't, can I change it?
- Will cooking odors come into this space, making me feel hungry and distracted?
- Is this space big enough so it won't get cluttered when I spread out all my materials?
- Is there enough light so I can read without straining my eyes?

Temperature

You'll want to be comfortable when you study. Being too cold will distract you; it's difficult to take notes with cold fingers. However, being too hot can cause heat stress, which can hurt your accuracy, speed, and mental sharpness. Plus, it makes you sleepy! For good studying, the best temperature is between 65 and 70° F (18 to 21° C).

To make sure your study space is a comfortable temperature, test out a few spaces. Sit down and read or study for a half-hour. Are you under an air conditioning or heating vent that will make you too cold or too hot? Are you near a door that causes a draft whenever it's opened? These factors are out of your control and should disqualify a potential study space.

Surroundings

Your study space should be inviting. You should feel good about yourself when you're there. A pleasant space can make you more alert. Here are some tips for improving your study surroundings.

- The right kind of background music can promote relaxed alertness, which stimulates learning. It also may improve your recall. In theory, if you always study biology with Bach in the background, you'll remember biology facts when you hear Bach. But be careful with music that is too loud or that will tempt you to sing along.

- Let the answering machine or voice mail pick up your calls, ideally in another room.

- Turn off the TV (or better yet, study in a room without a TV).

- Some people like white noise: a bubbling aquarium, quiet instrumental music, or even an electric fan. White noise blocks out other sounds without creating a distraction.

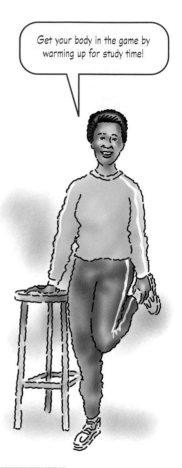

Get your body in the game by warming up for study time!

PRE-GAME STRETCH

Your brain is part of your body. If your body is uncomfortable, your brain has a harder time doing its work. When you're studying, you need your brain to focus on your work, not your aching back. You can stay comfortable by having good posture, avoiding eyestrain, moving around, and eating healthy snacks during long study sessions. (See *Fit for Studying.*)

FIT FOR STUDYING

Here are some ways to stay alert and be comfortable as you study.

- Sit up straight to keep your back and neck from getting stiff. It's worth the effort, and it can become a habit if you stick with it. Sitting up straight also keeps you alert and helps you concentrate.

- Make sure your reading material is propped up at a 45° angle from your work surface. And keep your eyes at least 15 inches away from what you're reading. If you're too close, your eyes can't focus properly. If you're too far away, you'll strain forward.

- Don't be afraid to get up and walk around every so often when you're studying. Stay in your study area, but try pacing around, doing jumping jacks, or performing simple stretching exercises. When you stand, 5 to 15% more blood flows to your brain. This means your brain gets more oxygen and is more stimulated!

- What about food? If you're going to study for more than an hour at a time, bring a healthy and easy snack, like grapes, so you can eat without mess or distraction.

THE WHISTLE: GETTING STARTED

Sometimes, it's easier to find a good study space than to actually sit down in that space and study! Getting started can be a big challenge.

The first step in meeting that challenge is planning ahead. Decide which tasks you want to accomplish before you sit down to study and develop a plan for accomplishing those tasks. The next step is breaking your big tasks down into smaller tasks. Several small tasks will seem easier to accomplish than one big task. With each accomplishment, you'll become more confident, which will motivate you to keep going!

Have a Game Plan

Before you start a study session, plan it out. Have a goal for each session and a game plan for achieving that goal. Ask yourself the following questions.

- What do I want to get out of this study time?
- What do I need to learn from the material?

Skim the material you need to study and decide how much of it you'll really need to dive deep into and how much you can cover with just a few notes. Not everything needs detailed attention. That way, you'll spend your time wisely and get more out of studying.

Timing Is Everything

Choose your study time carefully. Try not to set aside time you usually spend eating or socializing for studying; you'll only think about what you're missing. This can be hard to do when you're a busy working student with a family. You might feel that you don't have any time when nothing else important is going on! But there probably are adjustments you can make to your daily routine. For example, if you usually spend 2 hours watching TV after dinner, try spending just 1 hour watching TV and use that other hour for studying.

Also, you should try to study when you are naturally more productive and awake. Some of us are morning people; others are night owls. If you tend to feel fresh and alert in the mornings, consider planning some of your study time then. If you're groggy and tired in the morning, but come alive when the sun goes down, evenings are probably the best time for you to study.

Set Attainable Goals

Breaking up big tasks is part of setting attainable goals. When you set realistic goals, you set yourself up for success. By taking small steps toward your ultimate goal, you get moving, which is the most important thing.

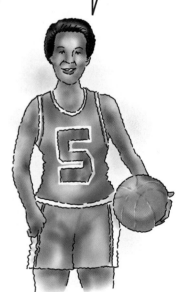

Learning to tune out distractions helps your concentration. Think of a basketball player tuning out a stadium full of people to make a foul shot!

For example, suppose you have a reading assignment that you don't feel like starting. Begin by telling yourself that you'll read for just 5 minutes, so at least you can get some of the assignment done. After the first 5 minutes, tell yourself that you'll keep reading for a few more minutes, and keep repeating this cycle. Before you know it, you'll have read for a half-hour or more, and maybe even completed a good portion of the assignment.

Other Ways to Get Your Brain off the Bench

Here are some more questions to ask yourself before and during study time to get your brain into study mode. These questions will help enhance your study time retention and later recall.

- Why is this information important?
- What does this information tell me about other topics?
- Is this information fact or opinion?
- What if I looked at this material in a different way?
- How can I compare and contrast different information?
- Does this material remind me of something else I've learned?

IMPROVE YOUR CONCENTRATION

We've already talked a little about the distractions that can interfere with your study time. There are external distractions, like smells or noises, which can cause you to lose your concentration. There are internal distractions as well, like hunger or anxiety, which can make studying difficult.

You can learn to improve your concentration skills so you can overcome those distractions. But it takes motivation to improve your concentration. You must want to learn the material in front of you. You have to know why it's important to your future career. Your desire to learn will help you stay focused on studying. Also, you need to be awake, alert, and prepared to learn. Being alert the first time you study helps you avoid multiple review sessions.

As an added bonus, improving your concentration during study time also helps you remember more material. This means you'll get better scores on tests, quizzes, and assignments.

DO YOU HAVE A WANDERING MIND?

Some people seem to remember everything they see or hear. Other people forget their own phone numbers. Does your mind wander? To find out how well you pay attention, ask yourself the questions below. If you answer *yes* often, you may have a wandering mind that could use some concentration strategies.

- Do you forget the names of people you just met?
- Do you ask people to repeat themselves?
- Do you lose track of what's going on around you?
- Do you sometimes stare blankly at a page?
- Do you sometimes feel like you don't remember information you just read?

It's normal for your mind to wander occasionally. But the most important thing is being aware of when it happens, so you can get back on track.

Find Your Focus

First, you'll need to prepare your mind and body to concentrate. The following strategies will help you find your focus before you begin studying.

- Take a short walk, about 5 to 10 minutes long, to clear your head and relax your body.
- Meditate for about 5 minutes. Sit quietly, perhaps in your study area with the lights off. Sit up straight and picture something still and peaceful. Breathe deeply and slowly.
- Try to avoid caffeine. Too much can cause you to become jumpy and make it harder to concentrate.

Concentrate!

Next, work on improving your concentration as you study. You can do this by using some of the strategies discussed earlier in this chapter, such as avoiding distractions and setting realistic goals. Here are some other good ways to improve your concentration.

- Study during a time of day when you're awake and alert.
- Focus on one topic at a time.
- Keep your brain active by engaging in different activities, such as reading, taking notes, and spending time thinking.
- Take short breaks every 45 minutes to 1 hour.

As with so many things, practice makes perfect when it comes to concentration. It might seem discouraging if you get distracted easily the first few times you study. But keep at it, and you'll train your brain to stay focused.

IMPROVE YOUR MEMORY SKILLS

Information is stored in different ways in your brain. That's why it's easy to remember some events or people and harder to remember others. Memory isn't a sense; it's a skill you can develop and improve. By understanding how memory works, you can learn ways to improve it.

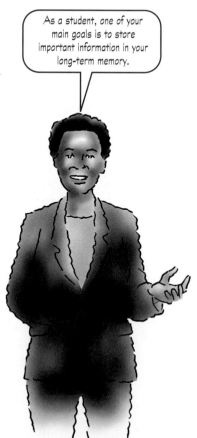

As a student, one of your main goals is to store important information in your long-term memory.

The Memorization Process

Why is it that you remember some things but forget others? It all depends on how the brain processes memories. The three stages of information processing are:

1. registration
2. short-term memory
3. long-term memory

As you learn new material in school, your goal is to get the most important information into your long-term memory. That way, you'll be able to recall what you learned during tests and put your knowledge to use later when you're on the job. Let's take a look at how memories move through the three stages.

Registration

During registration, the brain receives information. That information eventually may be understood and selected for remembering. Registration is a three-part process: reception, perception, and selection.

1. In the *reception* phase, you automatically take in information without knowing what it means. For instance, you might listen to a patient's bowels and hear whooshing sounds, without knowing what the sounds mean or what condition they represent.

2. During *perception*, you recognize what you've experienced and give it a meaning. Suppose you remember from class that whooshing sounds might mean the bowel is obstructed. You've attached a meaning to the sound—that's perception.

3. Finally, during *selection*, your brain chooses which pieces of information to remember. The information it selects depends on:

   - the information available at the moment
   - your reason for remembering it
   - your background knowledge of the topic
   - the content and how difficult it is
   - the way in which the information is organized

Your brain recognizes information as important or unimportant. If you decide something is important, like the fact that whooshing sounds could mean an obstructed bowel, then that fact is processed for remembering. If you decide it's unimportant, the information is forgotten. Processed information is then sent to short-term memory.

Short-Term Memory

Short-term memory can last as little as 15 seconds—that's short! Short-term memory can't hold a lot of information and what it can hold doesn't stay there for long. Research has shown that short-term memory can hold five to nine chunks of information, depending on how well the information is grouped.

For example, you can remember the numbers 1-9-2-9-0-0-7 by grouping them: 1929 and 007. 1929 is easy to remember because it's a date, and 007 is famous from James Bond movies. This way, instead of trying to remember seven different numbers, you only have to recall two groups of information. Grouping makes space for more data in your short-term memory.

> **BREAK IT UP**
>
> When you learn something new, it's hard for your brain to group the information because it's not sure of the relationships between the bits of material. You can make things easier on your brain by learning small chunks of information at a time, instead of one large chunk all at once. Your brain can organize small amounts of information more easily.

Long-Term Memory

After you've grouped information, your brain either forgets it or moves it to long-term memory, where it is organized and stored for long periods. How long depends on how completely the information is processed and how often you recall and use it. (See *Making Memories for the Long Haul*.) There are many ways to help move information from short to long-term memory, but the best way is to recall and use information immediately and often.

Getting Things Into Your Brain: Working Memory

The term *working memory* describes how your brain stores and retrieves information from short-term and long-term memory. Improving your working memory is critical to remembering what you study. You can use four strategies to improve your working memory.

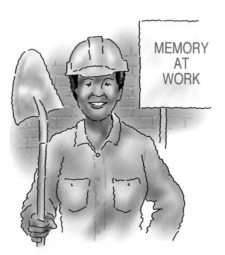

- selection
- association
- organization
- rehearsal

Selection

During selection, you single out the information you want to remember and start to select ways to process that information. For example, say you need to learn the steps involved in CPR. Because you know you'll need to demonstrate these steps in class, you almost unconsciously and immediately decide that all the steps are important to remember.

We make more conscious decisions about what is important all the time. For instance, a parent might know the phone number for her child's school or doctor by heart because she made a conscious effort to learn it. Why? Because she decided the number was very important and trained herself to remember it.

She selected the number as information important enough to go into long-term memory. Learning new material begins with making a conscious decision to remember it.

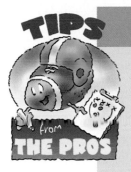

MAKING MEMORIES FOR THE LONG HAUL

There are many ways to make sure important information gets into your long-term memory. Use the tips below while you're studying to help you identify and sort long-term memory information.

Working alone:

- Attach strong emotions to the material you're studying.
- Rewrite the material in your own words.
- Build a working model of the material you're studying; create an image of it that you can remember.
- Create a song about the material or put definitions to a familiar tune.
- Draw a picture or create a poster using intense colors.
- Repeat and review the material 10 minutes after you read it, 48 hours afterward, and 7 days afterward.
- Summarize the material in your own words in your notes.
- Immediately apply what you've learned to activities in your daily life.
- Use mnemonics and acronyms to organize the material.
- Write about the material in a journal.
- State key information out loud, as though you were lecturing to a group of people.

Working with others:

- Act out the material or role-play a situation related to the material being studied.
- Join a study group or other support group.
- Discuss the information with a peer to gain an additional perspective and solidify the material in your mind.
- Make a video or audiotape related to the material being studied.
- Make up and tell a story about the material.

Association

Association is a very powerful way of committing something to memory. It involves making an association between something you already know and the thing you're trying to learn.

For example, to remember information about a particular disease, try associating that information with someone you know who has the disease. This will provide a memory cue that helps you recall the information later.

Organization

During organization, you memorize information in an ordered way. For example, if there are too many steps involved in CPR, break the process down into smaller chunks made up of a few steps each. With repetition, you can push each chunk, or group, of steps into your long-term memory. Rewrite the steps, recite them out loud, or act them out. This will help you remember the steps more efficiently, move them into long-term memory, and clear your working memory for the next piece of new information.

Rehearsal

An athlete may practice a certain skill over and over to perfect his technique. Think of a tennis player serving the ball again and again, going through the same motions each time. You can use a similar method to improve your memory skills. Rehearsal involves repeatedly reviewing information you've learned for short periods of time.

Several short bursts of rehearsal are better than one long cram session. For instance, rehearse the steps for CPR for 15 minutes four times a day rather than for an hour once a day. Challenge yourself to rehearse the steps at different times during the day, whether it's on the bus ride home, while you're making dinner, or while you're in the shower. Rehearsing information moves it into your long-term memory.

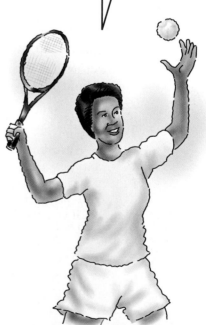

When it comes to rehearsing information, think of a tennis player practicing his serve over and over. With frequent rehearsal, the information you're trying to remember will become second nature!

Memory Retrieval: Use It or Lose It

As you have seen, information you process might not stay in your long-term memory if you don't use it regularly. It also can be forgotten if you're not interested in the information, if your purpose for learning is not strong, or if you have few or no connections between the memory and other pieces of information.

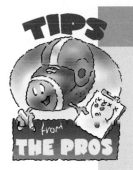

HUNTING DOWN A MEMORY

The next time you have trouble remembering something important, try these strategies to search for your lost memory.

1. Say or write down everything you can remember about the information you're seeking.

2. Try to recall events or information in a different order.

3. Recreate the learning environment or relive the event. Include sounds, smells, and details about the weather, objects, or people who were there. Try to recapture what you said, thought, or felt at the time.

Show Your Interest

In general, the more you care about a topic, the stronger your memory of it will be. For example, if you know you have a quiz next week on a particular topic in anatomy class, you'll store information about that topic in your long-term memory.

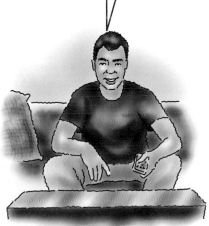

It's easy to remember facts about your favorite sports team. The more interested you are in a topic, the better your retention of it will be.

Understand It

You actually can memorize information without understanding it. Most of us know the words to the Pledge of Allegiance or the national anthem, but many of us do not know what those words really mean. But you have to understand a concept to be able to remember and apply it. Try putting new concepts into your own words and explaining them to someone else. If you can make a layperson understand it, you've got it.

Go Deep!

The more deeply the brain processes a topic, the more solid the long-term memory of that topic becomes. Processing depth depends on how you process the information, as well as your:

- background knowledge
- desire for learning
- intended use of the information
- level of concentration
- interest in the topic
- overall attitude

USE STUDY STRATEGIES

There are many study strategies that can help you recall information later during tests and clinical exercises. You've already read about a few of these strategies. Using a variety of study methods helps your brain take in and store the same information in different ways. This creates multiple pathways for your brain to use when you're trying to recall the information later. So give your brain a boost and see which study strategies work best for you!

Practice, Practice, Practice!

Practice and repetition are very similar to rehearsal. Practice not only helps you store information in your long-term memory, it also helps you retrieve that information from your memory when you need it. Here's how you can apply the strategy of practice and repetition as you study.

- Repeat information out loud or in a group discussion.
- Write or diagram the same material several times.
- Read and then reread information silently.

Take Breaks

Spaced study is a method that allows you to alternate short study sessions with breaks. Study goals are set by time or task. For example, you could read for at least 15 minutes or read at least three pages at a time. After meeting your goal, you would take a 5- to 15-minute break.

Spaced study works for several reasons.

- It gives immediate rewards for your hard work.
- It helps you complete manageable amounts of work.
- It helps you set deadlines so you can make efficient use of your study time.
- It keeps information moving from working memory to long-term memory. (See *Getting Things Into Your Brain: Working Memory.*)

- It gives you study breaks to keep you sharp when you're studying complex subjects.

Make Associations

Making links between familiar items and new information you want to remember is called developing associations. Once you establish them, these links become automatic. Each time you recall a familiar item, you also remember the information you associated with it.

Follow these steps to form associations as you study.

1. First, select the information you want to remember. For example, suppose you want to remember information about osteoporosis, a condition that causes a person's bones to become brittle.

2. Next, create an association to the information. To remember facts about osteoporosis, you might associate that information with a person you know who has the condition. (Osteoporosis reminds me of Mary, who broke her hip. Osteoporosis → Mary → brittle bones.)

To really work, associations have to be personal, such as associating a song, a person, or a scent with the item you're trying to commit to memory. You probably know certain songs that take you right back to where you were when the song was popular. Associate information to that song, and your memory of the information will be just as sharp.

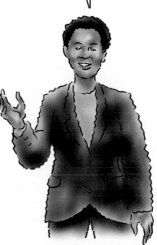

Have fun with it! Use acronyms and acrostics to enhance your long-term memory.

Acronyms and Acrostics

Acronyms and acrostics are handy for recalling information, too. Acronyms are created from the first letter of each item on a list. *ASAP* is an acronym for the phrase "as soon as possible." The acronym *HOMES* helps people remember the Great Lakes:

H Huron

O Ontario

M Michigan

E Erie

S Superior

Acrostics are phrases or sentences that are created from the first letter of each item in a list. In health care, a well-known acrostic is one about the 12 cranial nerves: *On Old Olympus' Towering Tops, A Finn and a Swedish Girl Viewed Some Hops.* This stands for the olfactory, optic, oculomotor, trochlear, trigeminal, abduscens, facial, sensorimotor, glossopharyngeal, vagus, spinal accessory, and hypoglossal nerves.

Acronyms and acrostics work in situations where it's hard to find a personal memory or other association for a piece of data. (For example, it's difficult to feel personal about the 12 cranial nerves.) Acronyms and acrostics associate key information to a new but easily remembered word or phrase, improving your memory of the information.

Put Information in Its Place

You can understand a piece of information more easily once you're able to put it in a larger framework of understanding. For example, a small area on a street map makes more sense when you're able to view the map in its entirety. Sometimes, it helps to see how the information you're studying fits into the bigger picture.

You can apply this practice to studying by learning more about a topic in general before focusing on a particular assignment. Television programs, videos, or magazine articles are good places to look for general information. After you've gained some background knowledge of a certain topic, you'll be able to associate new information about that topic with what you already know. Your brain can then find a place for the new information in your memory.

Reduce Interference

Interference sometimes occurs when you're trying to remember two very similar pieces of information. It's like what happens when you tune in one radio station and another station's signal causes static, interfering with your reception. Your brain has to recognize the differences between the two pieces of information before you'll be able to commit both to memory.

For example, if you're trying to learn a lot of new terms and two of them are similar, you might have trouble remembering either of them. To reduce interference, try to relate each new term to information you already know. Your background knowledge will help you recognize the differences between the two terms, allowing you to store each as a separate memory.

If you need to study similar subjects one after the other, take a break between study sessions. Moving to a different study space or changing positions will make your brain aware that there is a difference between the

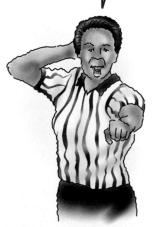

Interference! Two similar pieces of information may interfere with your brain's ability to remember either of them. Focus on what makes each item different.

two subjects. It will associate one subject with one location and the next subject with the next location. This way, your brain can better organize the new information in your memory.

Create Lists

Lists are another well-known study aid. You can organize ideas by categories that they have in common. The point is that you create a classification system of some kind. Because items relate to each other within the system, you can rearrange and reorganize that information as needed to help your recall.

For example, suppose you're learning about different types of drugs in your pharmacology course. To help you study the material, you could create lists of drugs according to what they're used for. Drugs used to treat diabetes would form one list, while drugs used to treat heart conditions would form another, and so on.

Use Imagery

People often think visually—in images instead of words. Visual aids can help you recall familiar and unfamiliar information when you're studying. This is because images are stored differently than words in the brain. Adding meaningful doodles, colors, or symbols to your notes allows you to organize them visually by topic. When you use visual representations effectively, you'll remember more information with less effort.

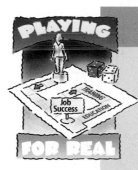

VISUALIZE IT!

I'm Chantal. I used to have a real mental block when it came to the forearm bones. I just couldn't remember which one was the radius. Then I figured out how I could use imagery to help me remember. I pictured myself taking a patient's radial pulse—the end of the radius is located right beneath that pulse! Now, when I have to know the forearm bones, I just picture taking a pulse. The image in my head helps me remember which bone is the radius.

Think in Pictures

Imagery helps you link concrete objects with images, like a picture of a tree with the word *tree*. It also links abstract concepts with symbols, like a heart shape for *love*. As you study, draw pictures or symbols to illustrate important concepts. These visual cues will give your brain yet another way to remember the information.

Red Card!

In sports, colors can have meaning. Soccer fans know that a yellow card indicates a penalty, while a red card gets the offending player sent off the field. Colors can give meaning to the information you're studying as well. For example, you could use a variety of highlighters to color-code your lecture notes according to topic. You also could use color to indicate key points or to mark two or more related concepts in your textbook. Using color gives you a way to visually organize the material you're trying to learn and remember.

IMPROVE YOUR EFFICIENCY

There are many ways to improve your efficiency as you study. Most of these techniques focus on helping you restate material in your own words. Here, we'll look at *reciprocal teaching* and *metalearning*.

Reciprocal Teaching

Reciprocal teaching is a method that will help you:

- summarize the content of a passage
- ask one good question about the main point of a passage
- clarify difficult parts of a passage
- predict what information will come in the next passage

Reciprocal teaching starts when you and the instructor read a short passage silently. Then, the instructor summarizes, questions, clarifies, and predicts based on the passage. Next, you read another passage, but this time you do the summarizing, questioning, clarifying, and predicting. The instructor may give you clues, guidance, and other encouragement to help you master this method.

You can take the reciprocal teaching method into your individual study time after you've practiced it with an instructor. Read a passage or section, then summarize, question, clarify, and predict based on the passage. When you're done, you'll know the material inside and out.

Reciprocal teaching helps the student become the teacher.

Metalearning

The prefix *meta* means something that is aware of itself and refers to itself. Metalearning is a process where you ask yourself questions to become aware of your own motives, understanding, challenges, and goals.

In metalearning, you ask yourself a series of questions.

- *Why am I reading or listening to this?* In the metalearning process, you briefly state your purpose for studying certain material. Your purpose and goals set the stage for your study time.

- *What's the basic content of this material?* Preview material before you read. For long or complex material, translate your preview into a chapter map or outline. You also might want to write what you know about the topic and what you'd like to know or think you will know once you're done studying.

- *What are the orientation questions?* Orientation questions give background information on a topic or concept by asking about definitions, examples, types, relationships, or comparisons. The purpose of using orientation questions is to see how many questions you can ask about the material and how many answers you can find.

- *What's really important in this material?* Identify information you should focus on, ignore, or just skim. As in planning ahead, this helps you figure out where to spend your time. If you can't decide whether something is important or whether it should be skimmed or ignored, assume it's important.

- *How would I put this information in my own words?* Putting things in your own words is called paraphrasing. Paraphrasing helps you understand concepts better and identify gaps in your learning right away. Make sure you can put unique terminology for each subject into your own words.

- *How can I draw the information?* Visual learners can get a lot out of drawing the information they're studying. Representing information in pictures is very useful for building understanding.

- *How does the information fit with what I already know?* If you already have a solid foundation of knowledge about a topic, you can learn new things about that topic more easily.

REST, RELAX, AND EAT RIGHT

As you study, your brain needs time to sort information and store it in your memory. To do that, your brain needs rest. Have you ever had a busy day at work and then dreamt about doing the same tasks? It's no accident. During deep sleep, the brain keeps right on sorting and storing information, saving important information and forgetting unimportant details. By getting enough rest and relaxation, your brain can take a break from processing information, allowing it to catch up.

As you learned in Chapter 4, what you eat also has an effect on how your brain functions. A healthy, balanced diet will give you the energy and nutrition you need for studying.

REWARD YOURSELF

After studying, reward yourself for a successful study session. The reward can be something small, such as allowing yourself to watch an extra half-hour of television in the evening. The reward itself isn't important, as long as it's appropriate in size to the task you completed. What's important is that rewards give you a good feeling about the work you've done. And a positive attitude toward studying, as you learned earlier in this chapter, will motivate you to keep at it!

The Importance of Networking

We've all heard of networking, but what is it? In Chapter 2, you learned about the concept of networking in terms of forming study groups. Here we'll explain the importance of tapping into the knowledge of others *and* contributing to the knowledge pool—a win-win situation.

THE HOME TEAM: WHAT IS A NETWORK?

You've heard of television networks and computer networks. A network is an interconnected group or system. A television network is a group of local stations that share the same programming. A computer network is a group of computers that share information. A network can be big or small.

A network also can be a group of people who choose to share information and expertise with one another. Usually, people "network" with others who share their interests or occupation. A network has several key features.

- It is voluntary—you choose to join and participate in a network.

- It is focused—information and expertise on a specific topic are shared.

- It is respectful—members all treat each other with respect, sharing ideas and asking questions freely.

Sometimes, a network forms naturally. For example, your instructor might put you into a group in class. You might find this group stays together even after the course is over. But usually, networks have to be purposely created.

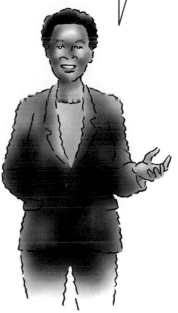

Your network is your home team—it's easier to succeed when you work together!

HOW TO CREATE A NETWORK

Creating a network requires three things.

- You have a reason for forming the network. That way, you can keep the network focused.

- You add value to the network. You can contribute information as well as consume it.

- You have ground rules for participation.

Creating a network takes time, but it's worth it. If you develop a network of people you know and like, who can help you *and* learn from you, then you'll get the full benefit of this kind of interaction. Learning how to network successfully is very important for your future career, when you'll need to keep up on the latest information and techniques.

First-Round Draft Picks

Begin by making a list of some classmates you'd like to include in your network. Choose two or three people from that list. Your network can grow over time, but it's best to start small. You'll find it's easier with a small group to get to know everyone and to arrange times to meet.

To narrow your list, think about the people on it.

- How much time does each person have to spend?

- How might each person contribute?

- What are people's strengths and weaknesses?

- Have you ever worked together before?

Weaknesses don't necessarily disqualify someone—we all have them. But think about how that person will fit into the group.

Setting Up the Rules

Once you have your list, approach the people on it and suggest networking. The key here is to be clear about what you're proposing and to be respectful. If you want to have an informal network, where members e-mail when they have a question or something to contribute, explain that. If you want a formal network, where members meet regularly in addition to e-mailing and having one-on-one conversations, make that clear.

Remember to be open to the suggestions and constraints of others. If someone can't meet when you'd like, but she's very valuable to the network, be flexible so you can include her. If someone doesn't have the time or simply doesn't want to be part of a formal network, graciously thank him and let him off the hook. He can still be a personal, one-on-one source of information and sharing for you.

HOW TO USE A NETWORK

Remember, networking means interaction. Everyone in the network contributes information *and* consumes it. That's what makes the network valuable; everyone benefits from everyone else's knowledge and different ways of looking at things. When you network, you share what you know with others who do the same, creating something new in the combination of ideas. It's the sharing of ideas, or the dialogue, that makes a network successful.

Give Credit Where Credit Is Due

Information shared in a network is free. If something is shared in a network, all the members of the network should be allowed to use the information. But that doesn't mean you write down what someone else says and pass it off as your own opinion or knowledge. Always acknowledge your network. Be honest by saying your idea was inspired by someone in your network.

Network Members Are Study Partners—Not Accomplices!

A network is great for helping you study. But be vigilant about keeping your group on the up and up. If someone in the network offers to share quiz answers with you after the quiz, that's great. But if it's *before* the quiz, that's a red flag. Members of a network shouldn't ask for answers to tests or special favors. They share strategies, ideas, and information.

Safe!

As you read in Chapter 2, once your main networking group is established, you're likely to
get people's home phone numbers and other
personal information, like e-mail addresses or
home addresses. Guard these carefully, and don't
share them with anyone
without asking first. And
remember not to wear out
your network with con-
stant contact, especially
with network members
who are busy with their
home lives and jobs.

> Be safe! Only give out your e-mail
> address and phone number to people
> you trust. And *never* share other
> people's contact information without
> asking first!

WHEN TO NETWORK

Informal networking goes
on all the time—between
classes, over lunch, and
on the phone. Activate your formal network at specific times:

- *At the beginning of the semester.* Find out which students
  in your class have had this instructor before and what
  you should expect. Ask them for tips and advice about
  being successful in this class, but *never* ask for old tests
  and quizzes.

- *After class or lab sessions.* Strike while the iron is hot.
  Talk about the ideas you had during class, find out what
  classmates thought, and then debate and expand the conversation. Take notes of your conversations next to your
  lecture notes.

- *After a missed class.* Call on your network to fill you in, but
  remember not to lean on your network to do your work
  for you.

Scheduling Meetings by the Book

It's great to have a regularly scheduled time for formal
networking—a time when everyone comes prepared to discuss
a certain topic. Meeting regularly to go over material helps you
all come up with new ideas and approaches.

It can be hard to find a time when busy people can meet. Do
the best you can to come up with a regular meeting time, such
as every week or every 2 weeks. If evenings are best, go with

that. If two half-hour meetings a week are better for everyone's schedule than one hour-long meeting per week, go with two half-hour meetings.

When You Can't Find a Scheduling Solution

If you are unable to find a time to meet in person with everyone, create an online group site or message board. Everyone can visit the group site and contribute to it whenever they're free. You can create a group on Web sites like Yahoo where members log in and talk via instant message boards. But be vigilant about keeping passwords strictly within the network, for safety's sake. You'll want to avoid having strangers posting on your site.

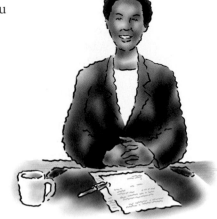

When participating in an online discussion, only talk to people you know and trust.

WHERE TO MEET

There are many places to meet. Finding the one that is right for you can take a little trial and error—what seems perfect before the semester begins may not actually work out. Keep at it until you get to the right place.

On Campus

Many students find it easiest to meet on campus in a common area or in a library discussion room (just make sure you're not out in the middle of the library disrupting others). If your regular meeting time falls during the school day, this may be the best option for you.

Off Campus

Meeting off campus may work better if your meeting time falls after classes have ended for the day. It also may work better for members who are not on campus (professionals in the workplace or students at another campus). In this case, meet at a centrally located coffee shop or take turns hosting the group at your homes. Just remember—safety first! Make sure you know everyone in your group well before you agree to meet them somewhere or invite them to your home.

Online

You also can network online, as mentioned previously. This works well for a network that is spread out. For instance, if your cousin is a health professional in another state, he can be included in an online network. Just remember to be careful online. All the rules for face-to-face networks apply here. Only talk online with people you trust and don't invite strangers in without talking with the whole group first. Avoid giving out network members' e-mail addresses. You should only share information online with people you know and trust.

WHY NETWORK?

You've already seen many reasons why networking is valuable. Having a study group you can count on, getting tips for succeeding in a certain instructor's course, and being able to borrow notes from someone when you can't make it to class are all good reasons to network. As a student, networking gives you advantages you wouldn't have if you choose to keep to yourself.

But, perhaps the most important reason to network is to give and receive moral support. Your peers at school probably understand better than anyone else the challenges you're facing. Members of your network can offer support by:

- listening to your ideas
- sharing ideas with you
- making study time more relaxing
- helping you in tough times

Networks provide moral support by bringing people with the same goals together to help each other. The more you give, the more you get, and the better you feel.

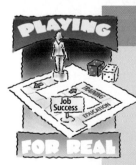

UNEXPECTED BENEFITS OF NETWORKING

Hi, my name is Roman and I'm training to become a medical coding specialist. I didn't like the idea of networking when I first started taking courses. It's hard for me to meet new people, and I usually prefer to work on my own anyway.

But when I started having trouble in my medical terminology course, I had to ask for help. My academic advisor suggested that I talk to some of my classmates and try to form a study group. It wasn't easy, but I introduced myself to a couple of guys in my class and we started meeting regularly every week. Not only did my grades improve, but I ended up gaining two friends—something I wasn't expecting at all!

Giving Your Two Cents

A good network listens to every member because every member has something valuable to say. Even though every member might not be an expert or have 20 years' experience, each person studies hard, makes the most of what he does know, and wants to learn more.

In a good network, all members share their ideas and information. No one should be worried that what he says will be taken out of context or used to try to gain an unfair advantage. No one tries to gain from other people's experience without sharing his own. In a good network, everyone contributes fairly and benefits equally.

The Huddle

A network should be made up of people you like and respect. A networking session should be stress-free and informal. You should be able to laugh, share funny stories, and confide your doubts and worries without being concerned that the whole school will find out about it later.

For example, a football player wouldn't leave the huddle to tell the other team what the next play is going to be. That would be disloyal to his teammates. Be sure to have the same respect for the other members of your network. If someone mentions a private concern to the rest of the group, avoid the urge to gossip. Keep private information within the network.

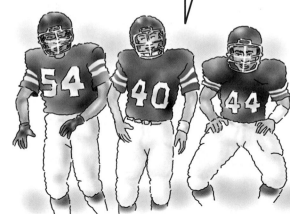

Teammates trust each other—be the kind of person your network can trust. If another network member mentions something in confidence, avoid the urge to gossip.

Resourcefulness

In this chapter, you've learned about studying on your own in a private space. This chapter has also discussed studying with other people in a network. Now, let's look at some other study resources.

Resources are any tools that help you study. They can be CDs, tutors, learning labs, videos, and even special seminars on improving your learning techniques. Most are free, and, once you get the hang of how and where to find them, you'll find that resources like these are invaluable.

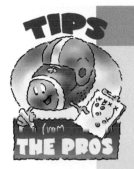

SEARCHING FOR RESOURCES: THE STARTING LINE

If you're having trouble finding out about the resources offered by your school, you probably just need to know where to look. Here are some tips to get you started on your search.

- Visit your school's information office and ask where you can find out about things like free seminars and learning labs.

- Ask your academic advisor to point you in the right direction. If you're struggling with a certain course, for example, your advisor may be able to suggest a possible tutor.

- Visit your school's Web site. You may find a "Student Services" section or a link to the Office of Special Services at your school and its list of offerings.

- Ask a librarian about resources available to students in the campus library. As a student, you may have access to special computer search engines, videos, and professional journal articles.

SEEK OUT FREE RESOURCES

Most schools provide a variety of free services to any student who seeks them out. It can take some hunting to find the free resources available to you. There are so many bulletin boards crammed with flyers advertising services and events that they can all merge into a senseless blur.

The fact that you also have to use your own initiative to find many free resources can be daunting. Who has the time and energy to track these things down? But, as usual, making the effort is worth it. Because so few students take the time to find all the resources available to them, there usually is an abundance of resources waiting for the person who does make the effort.

Some basic free resources you might find at school include:

- your instructor
- informal study groups
- your campus library

- learning labs
- special services, including the counseling center

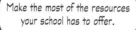

Make the most of the resources your school has to offer.

Help From Your Instructor

One free study resource is obvious: your instructor. Besides being available by phone or e-mail, almost all instructors have regular office hours when they are available to meet with students one on one. You can go to your instructor's office and go over anything you need help with. It's like having the instructor as your private tutor—for free! Find out when the hours are and put them into your schedule. And remember to share what you learn with your network.

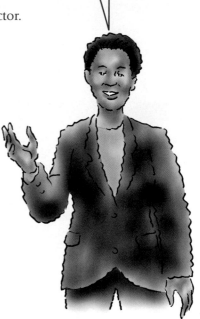

In the Dugout

Check your class syllabus to see if you need to make an appointment for one-on-one time with your instructor. Also, keep in mind that office hours are for everyone in the class. Your instructor will have limited time to help you during office hours. If you feel like you need more help, such as weekly, extended one-on-one tutoring, ask your instructor to recommend a personal tutor.

Other Ways to Communicate

There are other options aside from meeting your instructor in her office. Some instructors offer help over the phone or by e-mail. Some even set up online discussion boards. Remember not to assume that you can call your instructor at any time or that you can call as often as you want. Your instructor's time should be respected and shared equally with other members of the class. Be sure to call only during the appointed times.

If you send an e-mail, you may not get an answer immediately. Most instructors will tell you what their response time is for e-mail. Ask your instructor if she doesn't include this information in the syllabus.

Informal Study Groups

Often, members of a class form informal study groups. They get together before or after class to go over the material. These are drop-in groups where you are under no obligation to attend, though you are expected to contribute to the discussion.

If you notice students gathering after class, hang around and see what they're talking about. If they're going over class material, introduce yourself and see if you can participate, too. Just remember to apply the rules of networking here:

- no plagiarism
- no looking at quizzes or tests beforehand
- equal parts providing and consuming information
- never meeting someone alone whom you don't know well

Informal but productive study groups can turn into formal networks.

The Campus Library

Your campus library has a wealth of resources: videos, books, articles, and other supplemental materials. Find out if there's a free orientation tour on how to use the library so you know how to find everything you need. Knowing how to use the reference area of a library is invaluable, but you may need to ask for help to use it effectively.

Learning Labs

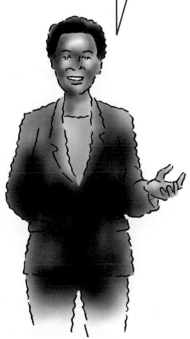

Find out whether your campus counseling center offers free seminars. There might be one that captures your interest!

Many schools have learning labs that are free for students to use. These labs usually have very specialized learning material in them. For example, there may be life-size plastic anatomical models to help you learn anatomy. Some will have computers to aid you in learning how to use certain software programs. Knowledgeable people who can help you make the most of these specialized resources usually staff learning labs.

Special Services

Most schools also are required to provide special services to eligible students with disabilities—but students generally must seek out these services themselves. Your school most likely has an office dedicated to helping students with special needs. Find that office to learn more about the resources available on your campus.

The campus counseling center is also a good place to investigate. These centers often sponsor free seminars on studying, how to stay healthy, and how to manage stress. These can be great places to pick up information to share with your network.

TEXTBOOK RESOURCES

Textbooks often come with CDs or workbooks that are loaded with practice quizzes, sample test questions, games, and other learning tools. By taking advantage of these resources, you will be way ahead of the competition come test time! Textbook publishers also often have Web sites where you can find lots of resources to help you study. Your textbook may have a toll-free phone number in it that you can call for help with finding supplemental materials.

THE WONDERFUL WORLD WIDE WEB

As you learned in Chapter 5, you can find a wealth of supplemental material online for any course you're taking. Just remember to be safe.

- Make sure Web sites are trustworthy. Web sites that end in .gov or .edu generally contain reliable information.
- Make sure any Web site you use is accurate (up-to-date and unbiased). Personal Web sites, like blogs, may have a lot of information, but there is no guarantee that the information is accurate.
- Make sure the Web sites you use are free.
- Make sure you don't have to give out your own personal information to use a Web site.
- If possible, get a list of reliable Web sites from your instructor.

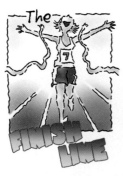

- Look at things, such as the lighting, temperature, and surroundings, when considering a possible study space.
- Set goals for each study session to give yourself a game plan to follow and to make the most efficient use of your study time.
- Get more out of studying by using strategies to improve your concentration and memory.
- Use different study methods, such as repeating information, taking short breaks, and using acronyms or acrostics.
- Study more efficiently by being aware of your own motives, understanding, challenges, and goals.
- Rest, exercise, and proper nutrition will give you the energy you need to stay alert and focused as you study.

- Networking is important because it allows you to share your ideas and learn from others. Networks also can be a source of moral support during the challenges you face as a student.

- Be a resourceful student! Seek out free resources offered by your school, use textbook CDs, and find supplementary material on the Web.

Review Questions

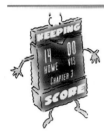

1. Name at least three different study strategies.
2. What are several challenges you might face when creating a network?
3. What are some examples of red flags that reveal an unreliable Web site?

Chapter Activities

1. Study Space Checklist
   - Review *Scope out a Study Area* and make a checklist of what your perfect study space would have.
   - Now, choose three or four characteristics that you can work on and create a to-do list to get them done.
2. Networking Exercise: Talk with at least two friends at school about creating a network. Each of you will then come up with one other person you know and trust from one of your classes. Give yourselves a week to contact the other people. Then, meet as a group to see how you all get along. If everyone seems like compatible network members, decide on a place and time to meet regularly.

Chapter 7

INSIDER TEST-TAKING TIPS

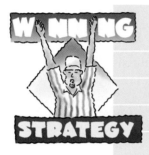

- Take care of your mind and body to reduce the amount of stress you feel

- Review the physical and mental signs of stress

- List common characteristics of anxious students

- Fight test anxiety

- Prepare and study for tests

- Use different strategies to do well on objective, subjective, and other tests

Does anyone you know *love* taking tests? Probably not! Tests are something all students face, and tests cause almost everyone anxiety. In this chapter, you'll find out how to plan and prepare for tests so you can improve your test-taking abilities and feel more confident. You'll also learn about special skills for managing test anxiety.

Health and Stress Management

Doing well on a test starts long before you take out your pencil on the big day. It starts with how well you take care of your mind and your body. Yes, studying is certainly key to your success, but how you care for your health and how you manage stress are very important, too.

Here's a quick review of what you learned in Chapter 1 about caring for your body.

- Regular exercise can lower stress, keep you fit and looking good, and make you feel better mentally and physically.

- Sometimes, rest is more important than completing every task on your daily to-do list.
- A balanced and nutritious diet is important for your health and managing stress.
- Breathing and relaxation techniques or yoga can help release tension.

In Chapter 1, you also learned that your mind needs recharging. Here's a review of some of the techniques you can use:

- *Keep negative thoughts under control.* Use positive imagery to move your mind toward your goals and away from your fears.
- *Calm your body to calm your mind.* When you have negative thoughts, use body-calming techniques (such as those discussed in Chapter 1) to put yourself in a more calm and relaxed state of mind.
- *Visualize yourself achieving your goals and overcoming obstacles.* Think about how you feel when you visualize these things and remember that feeling when negativity rears its head.
- *Build a social support network.* Family, friends, classmates, coworkers, and people who share your interests are all good choices for a social support network. They give you an outlet for discussing your problems with people who care for you and want to help.

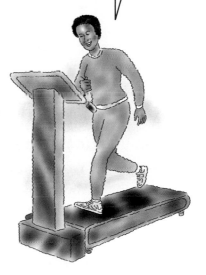

Running makes me feel tired right now, but later it will give me the energy I need!

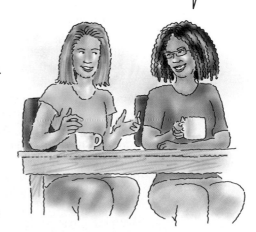

My friends help me see my problems in perspective and find solutions to them.

TEST ANXIETY

Remember what *eustress* means? That's right—good, or healthy, levels of stress. But most of us are more familiar with *distress*—high, unhealthy levels of stress. Most students experience a certain level of stress at test time, but for some, increased stress at test time interferes with their ability to think. They know the material. They've studied hard and effectively. They just get so tense at test time that they can't put down the right answers. The way to beat test anxiety is to first recognize it, and then prepare to fight it!

Are You an Anxious Student?

Part of recognizing test anxiety is figuring out whether you're an anxious student. The following sections describe several different characteristics of anxious students.

Feelings, Too Many Feelings...

Really anxious students go back and forth between focusing on new material and thinking about how nervous they are. They find it difficult to maintain their concentration during a lecture or a reading session. They keep noticing their discomfort and think, "I'm so tense—I just can't do this!" Because the very anxious student's attention is focused on worrying about doing a bad job, being criticized, or feeling embarrassed, she may miss the information she's supposed to learn.

Lost in the Details

Anxious students often have poor study habits. It's hard for them to learn if the material is:

- disorganized
- broken down in many parts
- difficult to understand
- focused on memorization

In these situations, anxious students are very easily distracted by irrelevant or minor details of the tasks at hand. They can't see the forest for the trees, which means they focus on details and miss the main point.

Under Pressure

You've probably heard sports commentators discussing athletes who "choke" in high-pressure situations. A rookie quarterback might have a great season and then fail to do well in the playoffs. Similarly, anxious students often have the potential to do well on a test, but they lack the test-taking skills needed to overcome their anxiety. They "freeze and forget" in a testing environment, even though they might do just fine in a less stressful environment, such as class.

A Little Anxiety Goes a Long Way

You've read about what goes wrong for very anxious students. But a little anxiety can be a good thing. Slight anxiety can improve your focus and mental sharpness. It keeps you from feeling complacent, like you don't really have to try. But if you're consistently underperforming or feeling nervous and distracted, test anxiety is probably taking over.

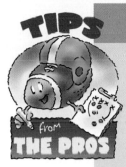

AVOID THE BIG FREEZE-UP

The most common test anxiety experience is a mental block, or "freeze-up." Though many students experience some level of this, students with severe test anxiety might read a test question over and over and never take in its meaning. Other symptoms of severe mental block are:

- doing poorly on a test after proving you know the material during class and in study groups
- feeling sweaty, shaky, or physically ill before and during a test
- fixating on how well you're doing compared with other students
- thinking about how to get out of finishing the test, such as by faking an illness

If you're so overwhelmed with test anxiety that you can't do well on tests—even when you've attended every class, studied hard, and proven that you know the material outside a testing situation—talk to your instructor about it. Your instructor might have another solution you haven't thought of. As an alternative, ask a peer tutor or friend to "test" you, with questions you haven't seen and a set time limit for completing the work. Taking practice tests beforehand can help you ease into the real thing.

Recognize Test Anxiety

There are many forms of test anxiety that come before and during a test. Here are some types of test anxiety:

- freezing up, when your brain doesn't take in the meaning of questions or you have to read questions over and over to understand them
- panicking about tough questions or about time running out before you're done
- worrying about the grade you'll receive
- becoming easily distracted, daydreaming, or thinking about how you could escape taking the test
- feeling nervous about your ability to do well or about how you'll do compared to others
- having physical symptoms of stress, such as sweating, nausea, muscle tension, and headaches

- feeling like you're not interested in the topic or like you don't care how well you do on the test

Prepare to Fight Anxiety

The key to staying on top of anxiety for most successful students is using a combination of techniques to prepare for tests. This section discusses tips and tricks all students can use. It's also important to remember that you need to prepare your mind and body. Keeping this balance will help you overcome your test anxiety and do your best.

Study Well

Studying well is the best preparation for a test—and the best cure for test anxiety. Studying can give you a sense of accomplishment that boosts your self-confidence. By knowing the material backward and forward, you won't feel as nervous going into the test.

Relax Your Mind

Relaxation, along with other stress-reduction techniques, can help lessen test anxiety. When your body is relaxed, your mind is free to absorb new information. Try using breathing exercises or meditation to clear your mind.

Think Positively

Test anxiety can be the result of low self-esteem. Focus on being positive about tests. Say to yourself, "I've studied hard and I know this material. I can do this!" Being prepared and having a positive attitude often lead to success.

Give Yourself a Break

If you start to feel anxious during a test, consider doing something to break the tension, such as putting down your pencil, closing your eyes, and taking a few slow deep breaths. If your shoulders are hunched, make a conscious effort to lower them and relax. If the instructor allows, you might even get up and sharpen your pencil or ask a question. Sometimes, you feel anxiety because you're physically tired and need a break.

Get Your ZZZs—Just Not During the Test!

Rest and relaxation are great fatigue-fighters. You can do more when you feel rested and relaxed than when you're tired. Try using these tips before your next test.

- Get enough sleep—at least 6 to 8 hours at a time.
- Change activities from time to time.
- Exercise on a regular basis.
- Relax by allowing yourself breaks for TV, music, friends, or light reading.

Sit Up Straight, Dear

Your posture matters when you're studying or taking a test. If you're sitting in an uncomfortable position, it stresses your muscles. This stress is communicated to your brain, which in turn creates anxiety. Slouching can hurt your back and make you feel tired. Sit up straight and allow your concentration to return.

Eat Well, Test Well

Good nutrition keeps you healthy. It also can improve your study habits and test-taking skills. Class time, work time, and study time often conflict with meal times. To counter this, avoid skipping meals and eat nutritious snacks between sessions.

If You Get Sick...

Even the healthiest person can get sick. When you're ill, you can't perform well on a test. So, if you feel very ill as a test approaches, contact the instructor. This shows you care about your performance and about missing the test. You may be able to work out an arrangement with the instructor, and this will help you avoid feeling anxiety about postponing the test. Be sure to follow all your doctor's instructions, so you can get well as soon as possible. Avoid using sick time as study time, and get the rest you need.

Make sure you eat breakfast on the day of a test!

Stay on Schedule

When a test approaches, keep things as normal as possible. If you normally take a walk before dinner, keep up with your routine instead of skipping your walk to study. If you usually sleep 8 hours a night, avoid the urge to cram until 2:00 AM. Breaking good habits will only contribute to your mental and physical stress.

Preparing and Planning Ahead

When it comes to test taking, preparation is important. Knowing *what* you need to do *before* you have to do it gives you time to work out the best *way* to do it.

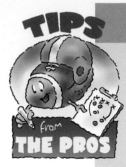

DEFEAT TEST ANXIETY!

Here's a checklist of things to do the next time you're feeling nervous about a test.

Before the test:

- Talk to your instructor and classmates about what the test will cover.

- Use the study skills you learned in Chapter 6. Develop a method that works for you!

- Divide your study time over several days instead of trying to review everything the night before the test.

- When studying, use all your resources, including your textbook, lecture notes, and completed homework assignments.

- Create 3 × 5 cards for each key concept or formula that might appear on the test. Then, use the flash cards to test your memory.

- Take a practice test. Find a room that's free of distractions and give yourself a specific amount of time to complete the test.

- Try to avoid studying right before taking the test. Put those notes away and take some time to relax!

- Arrive 5 minutes early so you'll be ready when the instructor begins the test. Just don't arrive too early—sitting in an empty classroom or listening to other students' nervous chattering might make you feel anxious.

During the test:

- Break the tension. If your instructor allows it, get up to ask a question, sharpen your pencil, or get a drink.

- Focus on tensing and relaxing muscles in different parts of your body, such as your neck and shoulders. Then, close your eyes and take a few deep breaths.

- Calm your nerves by putting the test into perspective. Life will go on after the test is over. Remember that doing your best is sufficient.

- Think of something calm and soothing when you feel test anxiety getting the best of you.

KNOW WHAT WILL BE COVERED

You can't study well for a test if you don't know what kind of test it will be. If you know what kind of test to expect, you can put your study time to good use. Objective tests, such as short answer, sentence completion, multiple-choice, matching, and true-false, require you to remember facts and details and to recognize related material. Essay and oral tests require you to make good arguments about general topics and to support your arguments with critical details.

Size It Up

To learn more about the test before you take it, attend class. Your instructor will probably explain the format of the test during class time. If she doesn't, visit your instructor during her office hours and ask these questions.

- Will the test be comprehensive or will it cover select material only (like a few chapters)?
- Approximately how many questions will there be?
- How will the questions be weighted? For example, will multiple-choice questions be worth 5 points each, while essays will be worth 20 points?
- Will the test require applied knowledge or basic facts?
- How much will this test count toward my final grade?
- What materials will I need? A calculator? Scrap paper?
- Will it be unusual, such as a take-home or open-book test?

Learn From the Past

If you've already taken tests in the course or attended another course given by the same instructor, you probably have some idea of what the upcoming test will be like. For example, you might know that the instructor focuses on details rather than principles or that he sometimes uses trick questions.

But if it's your first test for a particular course or instructor, you can still do a little extra preparation. Check for copies of past tests; your instructor may have them in his office, or they may be on file in the library reference room. Remember, past tests will give you an idea of what the test will be like, but you won't see the same questions on your upcoming test.

Learn From the Class

Think about how you've learned things in class so far. Which topics has the instructor spent the most time discussing? Have you focused on details or large concepts in class discussions? Some instructors offer review sessions before the test. If your instructor does this, be there and be prepared. Plan ahead of time for the review session by writing down the questions you'd like to ask.

GET READY, GET SET...

Give yourself a head start before you begin studying for an up-coming test. Thorough preparation short-circuits anxiety. Most instructors will give students a class schedule that lists test dates and other deadlines. Put those test dates in your yearly calendar. If your instructor didn't provide a class schedule at the beginning of the term, ask about approximate dates of upcoming tests.

Create a Game Plan

First, decide on an organized study plan. For example, you could set aside some time to study each day for a week before the test. Studying every day keeps the material fresh in your mind. Give yourself enough time to review your lecture notes, study materials, and old tests (if possible) several times. Choose a good place to study and perhaps a study partner. But even if your partner can't make it, keep the date yourself. Commit to studying and you'll be as prepared as possible for the test.

You might already review your notes after each class, which is good practice. But remember that it's not enough before a test. You'll need more intense review. In some classes, you may even have unannounced pop quizzes before a test. In those cases, you'll be glad you spent extra time studying!

The Trouble With Cramming

The trouble with cramming is that it doesn't work. You simply can't cram data into the brain and have it stick. Most of the information disappears in a few hours. And by the time you're sitting down to the test, your brain is so tired that it can't retrieve most of the data it did manage to retain. As a result, you "blank out" and are unable to answer questions you might otherwise have easily answered.

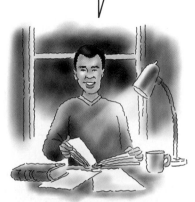

I can't cram in any more information—my brain is too full of fatigue!

Trying to Beat the Clock

When you have a test coming up and you feel un-prepared for it, the best thing to do is stay calm and focused. Double-check with your instructor or a classmate about the format of the test. Use your textbook to create a master study outline. Focus on chapter headings, summaries, highlighted words, formulas, definitions, and the first and last sentences of every paragraph. Write key points and an outline of each chapter on notebook paper.

When you're done outlining in this way, review your class notes and handouts. Make some "must-know" flash cards for what you feel is the most important information. Flip through the flash cards until you're too tired to continue. Make sure to wake up at least 1 hour before the test to review your outline and flip through the flash cards again.

Bring the Right Equipment

Next, remember to bring the right "equipment" to your study session. A student trying to study without a textbook is like a football player showing up to practice without a helmet! So, before you begin studying, gather all your review materials, textbooks, and notes. Look for information about the main terms, facts, concepts, themes, problems, questions, and issues that were covered in those materials. It's especially handy to compare the way your textbook covers an idea or concept with how your instructor covered it in class.

When you're studying for a test, try to avoid re-reading entire chapters of your textbook. Instead, armed with your knowledge about what kinds of questions will be asked and which topics will be covered, use your textbook's index and glossary to look up just those topics. Find definitions of key terms in the glossary and look for important details in handouts and other supplementary material. Make lists of definitions and rehearse them.

Make a Study Sheet

Summarize your notes on one piece of paper. Review this study sheet, then place it face down and try to recreate your notes from memory. Think about where each topic was placed on the page. That way, when you encounter a certain topic on the test, you can flash back to your notes page and actually "see" the information.

Equations and Graphs

For math or science tests, practice your skills by rewriting equations and graphs. Solve sample problems and write out formulas. If you have trouble with certain formulas or graphs, make a separate sheet for those troublemakers and review it during gaps in your schedule throughout the day.

Main Terms

For short-answer tests, go through your textbook or lecture notes and make a list of important terms. Then add the definitions and think of an example of each term that you could use in a short answer.

Practice Run

For essay tests, prepare by doing a practice run. First, look at previous assignments and tests to see how essay questions are worded. Then, choose a topic from the material you're studying now and develop an essay question. Finally, write an answer for your essay question, giving yourself as much time as you'll have during your upcoming test. (See *Subjective Tests* for tips on how to develop a good essay.)

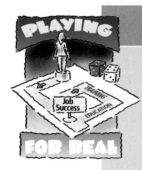

MY STUDY STRATEGY

My name is Sujala. I'm studying to become a pharmacy technician. When I have a big test coming up, I do a couple of things to prepare. First, I talk with the instructor and find out what kinds of questions the test will have—multiple-choice, short answer, or other kinds. Then I go through my notes and make practice questions out of them. For instance, I put my notes into multiple-choice format. That way, I can see how the information looks in test form. I make up a study sheet, too. The night before the test, I get a babysitter to watch my kids so I can review the study sheet and get it down pat.

Be Your Own Coach

Giving yourself a practice test allows you to be your own coach. Practice tests help you recognize the topics you struggle with most, which focuses your studying. To make a practice test, look at your study sheet and turn it into a series of questions. Then, answer the questions as if you are really taking a test. Sit in a quiet room and give yourself a certain amount of time to work. You may feel less anxiety when you take the real test if it feels familiar.

After you complete the practice test, use your study resources to check your answers. Spend extra time studying the questions you answered incorrectly.

Game Day

On the day of the test, there are several things you can do to make sure you're in top condition.

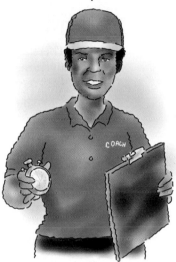

Be your own coach when it comes to studying! Give yourself a practice test to figure out how well you know the material.

- *Rest.* You need at least 6 to 8 hours of sleep the night before a test.

- *Eat small meals.* Breakfast is the most important. Just avoid eating too much, or you'll feel sleepy.

- *Avoid caffeine.* You don't want to be jittery.

- *Exercise.* Even a short exercise session will help you feel mentally and physically invigorated.

- *Have your test materials ready to go.* Do this the night before so you won't waste time frantically searching for something on test day. Include all written materials, notes, pens, erasers, pencils, calculators, and whatever else is allowed or required.

- *Arrive on time.* Make sure you wear a watch. Not only will this help you avoid being late or having to rush to be on time, but during the test you can track how much time is left. It's best to arrive 5 minutes early so you can be seated and ready by the time the test begins.

- *Pay attention to the test instructions.* Do this before you rush right to the questions. Read or listen to directions, such as "copy the question" or "show your work." Then, skim the test. Jot a few notes that bring bits of information to mind. By reviewing questions quickly in advance, your brain can work on answers to longer questions while you complete shorter questions.

- *Budget test time efficiently.* After you skim the test, think about how to budget your time. Think about how much time you have to finish the test, the total number of questions, the type and difficulty of each question, and the point value of each. If you start to lag during the test, don't stress. You can rebound by adjusting your schedule.

Test-Taking Strategies

You'll face many different kinds of tests during your student career, each of which requires unique strategies. There are objective tests, such as multiple-choice and true-false, and subjective tests, such as essays. There are vocabulary, reading comprehension, open-book, take-home, oral, and standardized tests as well.

You've probably seen some of these test types before. You might even have an idea of which kinds of tests are easier for you to take. But no matter where your strengths or weaknesses lie, all students can use the same basic tips to improve their test-taking skills. And once you can conquer any test, you'll be well on your way to success!

OBJECTIVE TESTS

There is only one right answer for each question on an objective test. The point is to test your recall of facts. Most standardized tests are objective:

- multiple-choice
- true-false
- short answer
- sentence completion
- problem-solving

When taking an objective test, look over the entire test to see how many questions there are. Try to answer them in order, but if you hit a difficult one, move on to the next. Just make sure you mark the tough question so you remember to come back to it. You can go back to the hard questions you marked when you've reached the end of the test and have extra time. Working on the easier questions first may help you answer the hard ones. Information from other questions might spark memories and prompt you to remember the answers.

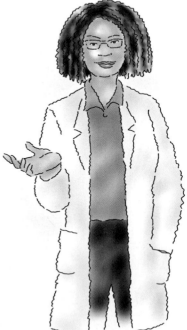

My "objective" is to succeed on any and every test!

How to Decipher Multiple-Choice Questions

There are certain guidelines to follow on a multiple-choice test.

- Read each question carefully. Phrases like *except, not,* and *all of the following* provide important clues to the correct answer.

- Try to answer each question before you look at the answer choices. Then, try to match your answer to one of the choices. Even if you feel you have a match at choice one, read the rest of the choices to see if there's an even closer match.

- Use the process of elimination to narrow your answer choices. Some answers are clearly wrong. Cross them out and focus on the ones that might be correct.

- Work quickly! You won't have time to go back and answer truly hard questions if you take too long checking and double-checking the ones you think you answered correctly.

WHO DECIDES WHAT'S *BEST*?

You do! Sometimes, test instructions tell you to choose the "best" answer. That means more than one answer choice is technically correct, but only one choice fully answers the question. You have to prioritize the answers to determine which best answers the question.

When you're prioritizing answer choices, use well-known theories or principles. For a question that asks what you would do first, for example, think of Maslow's hierarchy of needs. This theory basically says that while all needs seem important, they can be ranked. Needs at the bottom of the rankings can be dropped. In a well-written test, all answer choices seem plausible. No single choice stands out as obviously wrong. To apply Maslow's hierarchy to tests, you have to try and rank the choices. Look for a clue in the question that makes one answer better than the others. Sometimes, questions and answers are taken word for word from your textbook or lecture notes. If you recognize familiar words or phrases in only one of the options, that option is probably the right answer.

Be alert for "attractive distracters," or words that look like the correct answer but aren't. For instance, if *illusion* is the correct answer, *allusion* might be included as another answer choice.

True or False?

In general, true-false questions are meant to see if you recognize when simple facts and details are misrepresented. Most true-false statements are straightforward and are based on key words or phrases from your textbook or lectures. Always decide whether the statement is completely true before you mark it as true. If it is only partly true, then the statement should be marked false. Statements containing extreme words can be tricky. Watch out for words such as the following:

- all
- always
- never
- none
- only

Always watch out for statements with extreme words.

Short Answer: The 100-Meter Dash

Short answer questions are like the 100-meter dash of test items. These types of questions usually ask for one or two specific sentences, such as writing a definition or giving a formula. When you're taking a short answer test, organize the test items into three categories:

- answers I know without hesitation
- answers I can get if I think for a moment
- answers I really don't know

Answer the questions you know first, and then move on to the questions that need a little thought. Once you're rolling and feeling confident, go for the tougher questions.

Filling in the Blanks

Sentence-completion, or fill-in-the-blank, questions usually ask you to supply an exact word or phrase from memory. Sometimes, you can use the length and number of blanks as a clue to the best answer. Many instructors will indicate whether they expect one word, two, or a phrase by using longer and shorter blanks. Also, make sure the grammar is consistent. If you're really in doubt, go ahead and guess—you may receive partial credit.

Many times, the question itself will give clues to the right answer. For instance, a date may help you narrow the scope of answers by providing a historical point of reference. Suppose you think a scientific discovery might have been made by either Anton van Leeuwenhoek or Louis Pasteur and the date given is 1870. The right answer would have to be Pasteur, since van Leeuwenhoek died in 1723.

The Solution to Your Problems

Problem-solving tests are most often found in subjects dealing with numbers and equations, such as math and science. When you're facing a problem-solving test, first read through all the problems before answering any of them. Underline key words in the directions and important data in the questions. Make notes next to any questions that bring thoughts or data points to mind. Then, go back and begin to fully answer the questions.

What to Tackle First

Many times, students think they should start with the hardest problems so they can be sure those problems will be completed. They believe they can rush through the easy questions at the end. But it's actually better to start with the easy questions. They warm up your brain and build your confidence. Additionally, rushing to complete easy questions at the end can lead to careless mistakes and omissions.

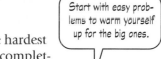

Start with easy problems to warm yourself up for the big ones.

Moving On

If you have trouble solving a problem, move on. When you come back to that problem, take advantage of the fact that you've been working on something different and look at the old problem in a new way. Will any of the strategies or formulas you used on the other problems work? There's usually more than one way to solve a problem. If the strategy you started with isn't working, try something else.

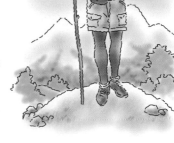

GET IT ALL DOWN

Show your work! If you make a mistake, the instructor will be able to see where you got off track and may give you partial credit. Also, when you write down all your work, you can check it yourself before you turn in the test. Checking your work helps you make sure you haven't made any careless errors or forgotten anything.

SUBJECTIVE TESTS

In a subjective test, there's no single right answer. Instead, you're graded on how well you demonstrate your understanding of the material. Follow these steps for successfully completing essay tests.

- Read all the directions, underlining important words and phrases.

- Read all the questions, even if you're not required to answer them all. Jot down facts and thoughts for each question.

- Estimate how long you think you'll need to answer each question.

- Choose the questions you want to answer.
- Outline each answer.
- Write the answers.
- Review and proofread your answers. Then, re-read the directions, making sure you followed them correctly.

Think about essays as endurance races. If completing a short-answer question is like running the 100-meter dash, then writing an essay can be compared to running a 5-kilometer race. It just takes a little more thought and planning.

Look Before You Leap

When you read all the directions in a test first, you reduce your chances of losing points by not following the directions. For example, the directions may ask you to provide three supporting facts for your statement. If you skip over that part of the directions, you might provide only one or two facts. When you're reading through the directions, underline the key points so you can refer to them with a glance as you write.

Duly Noted

Next, read through each question and make notes about any ideas or facts that come to mind. You can include things like formulas, names, dates, and your impressions. You'll need this information later as you create an outline. This step also helps you choose which questions to answer, since it gives you an idea of how much you know about each topic.

It's Just a Matter of Time

The next step is estimating how long it will take to answer each question. Consider things like the number of questions and how many points each question is worth. If one question is worth half your grade, for example, plan to spend half your time answering it. Factor in things like the time you'll need to organize an outline, write the essay, and proofread your work.

Organize an Outline

When you begin making an outline, start with your thesis statement. Choose a title that reflects your thesis and write it at the top of your paper. That way, you can use your title and thesis statement to guide your writing and keep it on track.

Content and organization typically count for most of your test grade. The five-paragraph format is a good way to organize your information. (See *Five-Paragraph Format*.) If you run out of time and can't finish your essay, you can at least turn in your outline to let your instructor know that time was the problem, not comprehension.

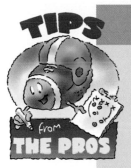

FIVE-PARAGRAPH FORMAT

The five-paragraph format is an easy-to-follow structure for stating and supporting an opinion. It's a great way to get started on your essay, and it also helps you finish writing by taking the guesswork out of where to go next.

1. *Introduction.* Briefly outline your opinion and the facts you will use to support it.

2. *First point.* State your first point and include one to two supporting facts.

3. *Second point.* State your second point and include one to two supporting facts.

4. *Third point.* State your third point and include one to two supporting facts.

5. *Conclusion.* Pull together the three main points in a summary.

Follow Your Game Plan

When you're writing, stick to your outline to avoid wasting time. Your thesis statement should be a clear, but brief, answer to the essay question. In your introduction, explain what the remaining paragraphs in your essay will discuss. The essay question may ask you to "explain a cause-and-effect relationship" or "summarize key ideas." Be sure to follow directions here.

Each paragraph in the body of the essay should make one point and support it with facts. This will help you be clear in your writing. There's no need to develop long, winding arguments. Go straight from point A to point B, and give the facts that led you there. Avoid making several points in one paragraph, or bringing in facts that don't really apply to your point or that you'll use later. Each paragraph should have a topic sentence that flows from your thesis statement. Write simple, direct sentences that follow one another logically.

In the conclusion, restate your thesis, then refer to the points you've made that prove it. Use the conclusion to draw your ideas together.

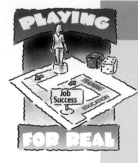

ESSAY TESTS MADE EASY

Hi, I'm Owen. I used to get psyched out about essay tests. I felt like I couldn't remember the main point I was trying to make—I got lost in the details. Now what I do is write my outline on a separate sheet of paper, and I leave a lot of space between sections. Then I write one sentence that gives a fact to back up my point under each section in the outline. After that, I go back and write one more sentence with a fact under each section. I do this until I have four sentences under each section. Then I copy what I've written onto my test paper, adding any more details I can think of. This way, I know my essay won't be top-heavy at the start and rushed at the end, and I stay on track with my main point.

Instant Replay

When you're done writing, go back and read the question you've answered and the directions again. Make sure you've answered the question fully. Then review your essay for grammar errors and make sure your handwriting is legible. Make corrections where necessary.

Using an outline helps you stay on track and prove your point in an essay.

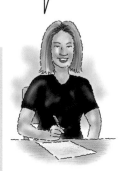

ESSAY QUICK-CHECK

After completing an essay, check your work. Ask yourself these questions regarding the following three elements of your essay.

Content:

- Did I stick to my thesis statement?
- Did I prove each point I made?
- Did I use examples?
- Did I distinguish fact from opinion?
- Did I mention any exceptions to my general statements?

Organization:

- Did I open with my thesis statement?
- Does the thesis statement answer the question?
- Did I follow my outline?
- Does my conclusion pull together all my points?

Writing mechanics:

- Does every sentence make a clear point?
- Did I use all words correctly?
- Are spelling, grammar, punctuation, and sentence structure all correct?
- Is my work neat and my handwriting legible?

OTHER TESTS

Other types of tests include:

- *Vocabulary.* These tests assess your ability to remember the meaning of a word and to use it correctly. They're used in foreign language courses or fields with specialized terminology.

- *Reading comprehension.* These tests will require you to read a passage and answer questions about its content.

- *Open-book and take-home.* You're usually allowed to use any and all materials you want when taking these kinds of tests. Critical thinking is more important than a good memory here. However, there's less slack given for making factual errors.

- *Oral.* Speaking clearly and fluently is key here. If you can choose your topic in advance, do so and prepare like you were going to write an essay, with a thesis statement and outline. Try to make three points supported by facts.

- *Standardized.* The GRE and SAT are two examples of standardized tests. They are used for placement and admissions.

Vocabulary Tests

Vocabulary tests call for some special strategies.

- Avoid decoy answer choices that look correct but aren't.
- Try to figure out if the word is a noun, verb, adjective, etc., and choose grammatically correct answers only.
- If you don't know the meaning of a word, try to remember where you've heard it and how it was used in the sentence. Select the answer that seems closest in meaning.
- Apply your knowledge of other languages. Prefixes, suffixes, and root words can offer clues about meaning.

Reading Comprehension Tests

These types of tests will go more smoothly if you read the questions first. Later, as you read the passage, you can focus on finding the information you need. Use only facts found in the passage! This is one case where applying outside knowledge is not helpful.

Open-Book Tests

Open-book tests require special strategies of their own.

- Use the index and table of contents to locate information.
- Avoid copying directly from your materials! Use as many resources as are allowed, but put ideas into your own words.
- Check your answers to make sure you didn't insert any incorrect information or unsupported arguments by mistake.
- As always, proofread your work!

Oral Tests

Oral tests should be prepared for like written tests, with one twist: you should rehearse your answers out loud. Here are more strategies.

- Dress well and look neat. Stand up straight and look your listener(s) in the eye.
- Speak clearly and speak up. Don't go too fast or too slowly (rehearsal will help you with this).
- If you're giving a speech, prepare notes and rehearse speaking with only a few glances at your notes. Never read directly from your notes—your voice will be muffled, and you won't make eye contact.
- Use your everyday language (except for slang) as much as possible. Using big or unfamiliar words will cause you to hesitate—and make mistakes.
- If you don't understand a question you get during or after your speech, ask for clarification. If you're still unsure, rephrase the question yourself.
- If you don't know the answer to a question, explain why. Perhaps it is outside your realm of expertise.
- When the test is over, gather your papers together and thank your audience for their attention.

Standardized Tests

Prepare for standardized tests by recreating the testing conditions and taking a practice test. Find a room that's free of distractions and allow yourself the same amount of time you'll have for the real test. The company who publishes the test most likely provides practice questions or other study materials. If not, there are often published guides, like books and software, for each test. These guides contain practice exercises and self-tests.

POST-GAME COMMENTARY

Reviewing your test after it has been corrected can help you learn where you got off-track and what you need to go over before the next test. When you get a corrected test back, ask yourself:

- Was there one concept or problem that tripped me up?
- How would I sum up the instructor's comments?
- Did I prepare adequately?
- Did I make any careless mistakes? How can I avoid them next time?
- What can I learn from my mistakes?

ONE FINAL STRATEGY

Tests give you an opportunity to evaluate how well you're doing in a course. Many instructors review tests with the entire class. One final test-taking strategy is to review your own test when it's given back to you. (See *Post-Game Commentary.*) Try to learn from the comments your instructor made. If you have questions, make an appointment to see the instructor during office hours.

Remember, it's never good to argue with an instructor about your grade during class. But if you have questions or believe the instructor made an error in grading, approach the instructor privately—outside of class. Be sure to present your concerns in a respectful way.

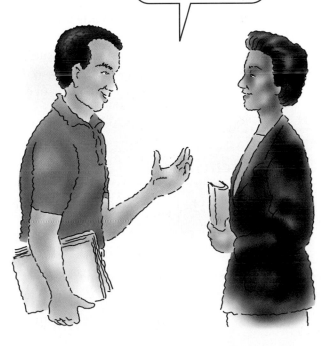

Try talking with your instructor to get more information on how to improve your test performance.

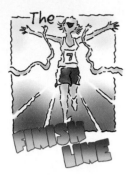

- Take care of your body by exercising, eating right, and getting enough rest.
- Meet stress head-on with relaxation techniques, positive thinking, and by relying on your support network.
- Studying, taking short breaks, making sure you're relaxed, and keeping to your normal schedule are ways to fight test anxiety.
- Give yourself time to prepare and plan for tests. Talk with your instructor about what to expect; create a study plan; and take practice tests.
- With all kinds of tests, always read the directions and skim through the questions before you begin.
- When taking objective tests, work on the easier questions first to warm up your brain and jog your memory.
- For subjective tests, create an outline to help you get started on your essay.
- Review all graded tests to see where you can make improvements.

Review Questions

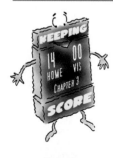

1. Short Essay: Write three to five sentences describing how to fight test anxiety

2. How can you find out more about an upcoming test?

3. Short Essay: Write three to five sentences describing how to write an outline for an essay and why doing so is important.

Chapter Activities

1. Exercise Checklist: Review *Health and Stress Management.* Choose the types of exercise and/or relaxation techniques you wish to do on a regular basis and make a note of what you'll have to do to get started.

2. Test-Taking Exercise: Divide into groups of three. Each group member will come up with a five-question test for this course. The questions can be multiple-choice, sentence completion, true-false, etc., or a mixture of

question styles. Arrange a time to meet for 1 hour. Each of you will take a test you didn't write and complete it in 20 minutes. For the rest of the hour, go over the tests as a group, helping each other see where you made mistakes or did well. Discuss the strategies you used to answer the different types of test questions.

MASTERING MATH

Many people have something we call "math anxiety." Perhaps the world of numbers seems strange and alien to them. Or maybe they had a bad experience with a math class when they were younger. It can be hard to overcome math anxiety, especially in a society where this anxiety is accepted as normal and understandable.

But overcoming math anxiety is important. Math is used in daily life, and math classes are unavoidable when you're in school. You'll want to be able to approach your math classes with confidence and a fresh attitude. Working through this section on mastering math can help you do that.

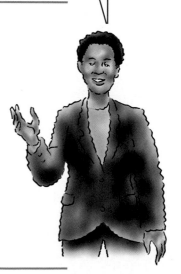

No matter where you go in your health career, you'll need good math skills. Take the time to hone them now!

Why Is Math So Important?

Many people struggle through high school math, hoping or assuming they'll never need to deal with it later in life. But math is all around you. Health care professionals need to be competent in math to perform many tasks:

- measuring solutions
- figuring dosages
- converting pounds to kilograms for weights
- creating department budgets
- scheduling staff assignments
- handling patients' claims and bills

Math Myths

One of the reasons it's hard to overcome math anxiety is that people believe things about math that just aren't true. Let's look at some of the most common math myths and how to shake them.

I'M JUST NOT GOOD AT MATH

People think of math as much harder than other topics, a kind of mystery where numbers are a foreign language. Sometimes, students are told they just can't do math and should leave it alone.

Are you a problem-solver? Are you driven to succeed? If your answer is yes, then you probably have greater math aptitude than you think. Math is all about solving problems. All you have to learn is the language of math—numbers—and you can start solving math problems.

MY CALCULATOR DOES THE MATH FOR ME

A calculator is just a tool to make math go faster. A calculator might be able to multiply more easily than you can. But it can't tell you what the x stands for in an algebra equation, or why an x is used in that problem in the first place. It can't explain what a square root is or how it's used in real life.

Think of your calculator as a tool to help you perform basics like addition, subtraction, multiplication, and division faster and with fewer errors. But be sure to learn how math really works. Your calculator can only take you so far.

I DON'T USE MATH IN MY LIFE—WHY LEARN IT?

Math is used in everyday life, even though you may not always see it or realize it. For instance, learning how to make conversions between different systems of measurement will help you calculate proper medication dosages for patients. Learning about other math concepts will allow you to create budgets at work and at home and complete many other vital tasks.

Success in Math Class

Some students dread math class. Somehow, they have the feeling they're supposed to know the material already. They're embarrassed to admit they don't understand a problem or a concept. But a math class is where you *learn math*. If there's any place in the world where you can put your math fears on the table and conquer them, it's math class. Here are some resources to use that will make math class a success for you.

YOUR INSTRUCTOR

Many students are embarrassed to tell their instructor they don't understand something. But your instructor is there to help you. If you hide the fact that you don't understand something, your instructor can't help you. If you let her know, she can.

A math tutor can give you the encouragement you need to keep working at it!

YOUR TEXTBOOK

Most math textbooks have plenty of practice questions, either at the end of each chapter or grouped together in the back of the book. Use these practice questions. Working through them helps you see some of the underlying patterns of a concept or technique and helps get you in the swing of using certain functions or solutions.

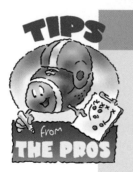

TIPS from THE PROS

PERSONAL TRAINER

There are people other than your instructor who can help you with math. You can find mentors at school or in your own family. And tutors are usually available—just ask your instructor or the secretary in the math department. Check bulletin boards in the math department and student centers, too; you'll probably find many ads posted that offer tutoring services. Some may even be free. There are also interactive online tutoring sites. So get off the bench and get some help tackling your toughest math problems!

WRITE IT ALL DOWN

Do each step of a math problem on paper, not in your head. Even if you know the formula well, write down each step. It helps you focus and gets your mind in the problem-solving groove. Just like a great musician still practices scales each day, you should write down even basic steps. It can also help you find careless errors in your work.

READ CAREFULLY

Get in the habit of reading very carefully when you go through a math problem. Most errors occur when you misread a problem.

Read through each problem out loud so that each part of it makes sense to you. Sometimes, you might think you see "add" when the symbol actually says "divide"; talking through the problem helps eliminate these kinds of errors.

SEE WHAT'S NOT THERE

If you don't understand the solution to a problem, there might be something missing from the problem itself. People make mistakes! Prepare a list of problems you are unable to work out, and discuss each one with your instructor. This way, you'll learn to see what you're missing.

DO THE MATH!

Students sometimes think that the assigned materials are the only ones they should use. But supplementary materials can give you fresh examples and practice problems. It's worth it to get these extra materials. Before you invest in one, make sure it has a lot of examples and step-by-step instructions. It should include proofs or derivations for the formulas it uses. Remember, different authors might use different notation systems, so be sure to familiarize yourself with them.

Preparing for Class

Math is sequential—every concept builds on a previous concept. If you miss one step, the next one won't make sense to you. That's why it's important to get to class and set aside time each day to go over what you've learned. Here are the basics to review daily:

- vocabulary
- basic formulas
- working cooperatively
- testing yourself

TALK THE TALK

Like many subjects, math has a specialized vocabulary. If you don't know the most common math terms, you'll have trouble with problems you could otherwise solve. Make a list of key words and study them. This list can include words emphasized by your instructor or your textbook, as well as words you find you have trouble remembering.

Treat math like a foreign language; you learn a language by picking up vocabulary words and memorizing them. You have to know how to pronounce vocabulary words, what they mean, and when they are used.

KNOW THE FORMULAS

Like vocabulary, math formulas form the basis for solving math problems. It's valuable to understand why a formula works the way it does. It's especially important to memorize basic formulas, as these are the formulas you'll use most often.

GO TEAM!

Usually, math isn't taught collaboratively. Students are rarely broken into groups to work something out. That's one of the reasons many students fear math: they are on their own, left to sink or swim.

But many instructors have come to realize the benefits of letting students work with a partner. Once you find a good partner, you can help each other solve problems. A partner can bring you:

Working as a team can help you tackle the toughest math problems.

- *Another point of view.* This helps you see more possibilities, thus improving your learning.
- *Increased personal accountability.* If someone is depending on you to help them study and learn, you will take that responsibility seriously.
- *An audience.* If you can explain a concept to your partner, you can explain it to the instructor on a test.
- *Praise and encouragement.* You and your partner will root for each other and provide positive feedback, helping create confidence.

PRACTICE TESTS

Take some practice tests to prepare for test day. Most textbooks offer practice questions. You also can find many Web sites that offer practice tests—some created by instructors for their students using old tests! Take the test without looking at the answers, and then grade yourself. You'll be glad you took practice tests when you sit down for your actual exam—they build your confidence and get you used to performing under test conditions.

Succeeding on Math Tests

Math questions generally fall into one of two categories: number questions and word problems. Both types involve solving problems and using math principles. Several strategies can be used to approach either type of test.

NUMBER PROBLEMS

Here are a few simple steps that can help you increase your likelihood of success when taking a number-problem test.

- Work carefully and deliberately. You can really sabotage yourself by being careless or working too fast. Thorough work is required. Write carefully, perform the calculations in reverse to check your answer, keep numbers in straight columns, and copy accurately.

- Write out all steps. Sometimes, students feel that showing all their work is childish. But it's a good practice at any age. If you write out your work, you can catch errors in it more easily.

- Estimate early. Try to estimate the answer to a problem before you start working. Then, solve the problem without referring to the estimate. When you finish your calculations, compare your answer with the estimate to see how close they are. If they're not close, you may have made a mistake in your calculations—a decimal point in the wrong place, an extra zero, etc.

- Make sure your calculations use all the information given in the problem. There's rarely unnecessary data in a math problem. Most of the time, each piece of data is essential to solving the problem.

- Read each question twice. After you think you have the right answer, read the question again. Have a checklist. Did you show your work? Did you answer in the correct units? Did you answer all parts of the question? Does your answer make sense? If your answers are yes, you're on the right track.

- Be persistent. Everyone gets stuck sometimes. There are ways you can get yourself moving again. Round fractions up

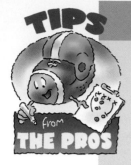

AVOIDING CARELESS MISTAKES

Careless mistakes are the result when students speed through problems. To avoid these mistakes and increase your accuracy, use the following tips.

- Write your numbers carefully so your sevens don't look like ones or fours and your eights don't look like sixes or zeroes.

- Whether you're doing simple or elaborate calculations, keep your digits in straight columns. You don't want numbers in the tens column being counted in the hundreds column.

- If you copy a problem onto another page, double-check to make sure you copied it accurately. You'd be surprised how often you can overlook a silly mistake—like writing a subtraction sign instead of a division sign—and not even realize it.

to whole numbers to put a problem into simpler form. Try to figure out what information you think you're missing. What doesn't make sense? Where do you lose track? If all else fails, move on to other questions and come back to the tougher ones later.

WORD PROBLEMS

Word problems have a bad reputation for being difficult. All word problems do is put numbers in a non-number context. There are some things you can do to make word problems more approachable.

- Look at the big picture.
- Plan well.
- Use strategies for dealing with difficult word problems.
- Learn from past mistakes with similar problems.

The Big Picture

When you're facing a test that includes word problems, look over the whole test first. As you read each problem, jot down notes in the margin about how you might solve it.

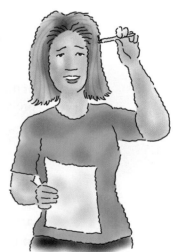

Work on the easiest problems first. Those are the problems where the solutions you should use are easy to identify. Solving easy problems first warms up your brain and builds confidence.

Set the Clock

Consider planning for the test as you would plan time for a study session. Allow more time for problems worth more points. Budget time at the end of the test to review and to go back to difficult problems.

Those tough problems can derail your planning, but it doesn't have to be that way. Stay calm. Try not to give in to panic or feeling overwhelmed. There are several strategies you can use to solve tough problems, including:

- marking key words and numbers, which can narrow the problem down to its essential elements
- sketching a diagram of the problem to make it more comprehensible
- listing all the formulas you think are relevant and deciding which to use first
- thinking about similar practice problems and how you solved them
- guessing at a reasonable answer if other strategies fail, then checking it. If you can't work out the problem to get to your answer, you may think of another solution.

Learn From Your Mistakes

After the test is over and you get it back from the instructor, read through the comments and suggestions. Try to avoid making assumptions about why you missed certain problems. Assumptions like "I just can't do math" or "It's just too hard" are unhelpful and counterproductive. Instead, ask yourself these questions:

- Did I make careless mistakes?
- Did I misread questions?
- Did I miss the same kind of problem over and over?
- Did I remember formulas incorrectly or incompletely?
- Did I run out of time?
- Did I practice enough, or did I skimp on practice problems?
- Did I let my anxiety get the best of me, making me miss problems I really know how to solve?

Based on your answers to these questions, you can identify ways to improve your performance on future tests.

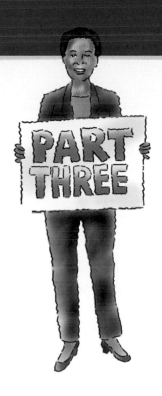

Game On

Chapter 8

CLINICAL ROTATION GROUND RULES

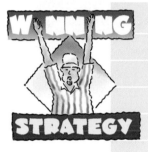

- Develop a plan to beat anxiety and stress
- Meet the standards of professionalism
- Preserve patient confidentiality
- Protect patient rights and safety
- Learn how to work in a culturally diverse environment
- Create a high standard of personal conduct
- Plan ahead for your clinical rotation

In this chapter, you'll look ahead to your clinical rotation or your externship—your first step toward a new career. You'll learn about the professional standards of conduct you'll be expected to meet and about the importance of protecting patient rights and privacy. You'll also prepare for handling changes in your schedule, and you'll learn how your clinical instructor can help you before and after you begin your rotation. This chapter will provide you with important information that will help you prepare for your clinical rotation and make it a positive experience.

Anxieties and Concerns

It's finally here: You're about to start your clinical rotation. You've often imagined yourself in a health care setting, putting your knowledge into action. You've looked forward to this day—and maybe dreaded it a little, too. It's one thing to read about the tasks you'll be asked to perform, but quite another to actually carry out those tasks in the workplace.

It's normal to be a little nervous about this step. It's a big one. But even though it seems like the unknown, remember that you *are* prepared. This is what you've been working toward every day. And you won't be alone. Your clinical instructor or clinical mentor will be there to help you.

Your clinical rotation is here—it's time to put anxiety in its place and get in the game!

YOU'RE NOT ALONE!

Although you're in a new environment, experiencing new things, you're not alone! Remember that all of the healthcare professionals you'll be working with were all novices at one time, too. You'll find camaraderie in sharing your experiences.

Your school may provide a clinical instructor to be with you during your clinical experience. Keep in mind that different programs may use different terms. Instead of "clinical rotation," you might hear the term "externship." Instead of "clinical coordinators," you may have "extern coordinators." Schools that do not send an instructor or coordinator to be with you usually arrange for someone on the job site to be your mentor. In either case, this person is there to help you and answer your questions.

PUT ANXIETY IN ITS PLACE

Whether you'll be assisting with patients in the examination room, working in a lab, or handling medical coding and billing, you probably have anxiety about whether you'll know how to do your job. That's normal. If you ask people who are already working in health care, you'll probably find they felt the same way when they started out.

It's important to address and deal with your anxiety. Mild anxiety probably won't affect your performance on the job, but high levels of anxiety will be a distraction. The following tips will help you put anxiety in its place.

- Use the relaxation techniques described in Chapter 6 to help relieve your anxiety.
- Make an appointment to see your clinical mentor. She can reassure you that what you're feeling is normal, and she

can help you identify your anxieties and come up with a plan to reduce them.

- Take advantage of the resources offered by your school. Many colleges also have counseling services that can help you cope with your stress.

SCHEDULE OUT STRESS

One thing that may be worrying you as you think about starting your clinical rotation is the demand on your time it represents. You've already pushed your schedule to the limits with school and work. Your clinical experience will bring about even more schedule changes. But you can manage these changes by knowing what to expect and how to prepare for them.

For example, do you remember the support network you read about in Chapter 1? Family members, friends, classmates, and coworkers can all be sources of encouragement and support during your clinical experience. If you accept help from others during this busy time, you'll feel less stressed. (See *Your Safety Net: Family and Friends.*)

YOUR SAFETY NET: FAMILY AND FRIENDS

Follow these steps to create a "safety net" of people you can rely on during your clinical experience.

1. Explain to your family that your schedule is going to change. Make sure they understand that this opportunity is important and that it's the next big step toward your new career.
2. Tell your family exactly what schedule changes are in store.
3. Offer concrete details about your new schedule.

   - If you have young children, talk with them about when or if they'll be in day care.

   - Talk with your family about which days or nights can be set aside for family time, such as family dinner nights.

   - Give specific jobs, like doing the laundry or helping out with other household chores to family members who can handle that level of responsibility.

   - Let your family know how much you appreciate their help!

4. Tell your friends about your new schedule, especially those you usually meet with for networking group, exercise, or other regularly scheduled events.
5. If you have roommates, make them aware of your schedule changes, especially if you do laundry

together, share the cooking or cleaning, or have other commitments.

6. Most importantly, let your family and friends know that they are important to you, and these extra demands on your time aren't permanent. You'll need their support to get you through the busy days ahead!

EMBRACE NEW SKILLS

Another thing that may be keeping you up at night is the thought of all the new responsibilities you'll have on the job. But the only thing that's really "new" about the tasks you'll perform is the fact that you'll be doing them for the first time in a clinical setting. After all, you've read about these tasks, practiced them in the classroom or laboratory, and you probably know just what to do.

Of course, knowing what to do in your head is different than actually working with a patient or staff member. That's why it's a good idea to practice your skills on fellow students or even family members, whenever possible. You will need to practice any skills involving needles and syringes in a supervised skills laboratory, of course.

During your clinical experience, you'll need a safety net. Let family members and friends help out from time to time!

Welcome to the Laboratory

Many programs require students to demonstrate certain skills in the laboratory before they're allowed to perform these tasks during their clinical rotation. If you know there are certain tasks you'll be performing during your clinical experience and you'd like more practice, use the skills laboratory to brush up on them. Most schools have times when an instructor or student mentor works in the skills lab and provides assistance. Take advantage of those times to get extra help.

Take the Plunge

Participating in skills labs will give you a good foundation for demonstrating skills during your clinical experience. Even so, it's natural to feel nervous the first time you actually have to do something in a real health care setting. You may feel like the only person in the room who hasn't performed a certain task a hundred times already. You might also feel like coworkers or patients are judging you unfairly for your inexperience.

The best way to get over the hump of hands-on experience is to jump in. You may feel awkward at first or reluctant to ask a question (especially in front of a patient or coworker), but with repetition you'll gain valuable practical experience very quickly.

> Jump right in! Experience will help you become more comfortable with the skills you'll use during your clinical rotation.

Personal and Professional Codes of Ethics

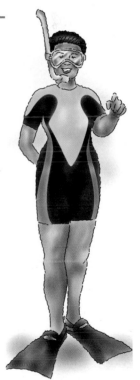

You're focused on acquiring information during your time at school, whether that means memorizing key terms, reading about difficult concepts, or figuring out how to apply your new knowledge. There's so much to learn that everything else seems like an unimportant extra. But there's one area that's just as important to your future career in health care—your code of ethics.

In health care, you're often entrusted with intensely personal information about people you don't know. You represent something to the patients you deal with—an ideal of a caring and educated health care professional. You're expected to be trustworthy and to take your job seriously.

You should do everything in your power to live up to this ideal. It may seem impossibly high, but it should be your goal. As you'll see, it's not about being perfect. It's about reminding yourself every day that what you do is not only special, but a privilege and a great responsibility as well.

A professional code of ethics addresses these areas:

- professionalism
- confidentiality
- patient rights and safety
- cultural diversity
- personal conduct

PROFESSIONALISM

The first item in the professional code of ethics is professionalism itself. Professionalism means:

- maintaining professional conduct while in the clinical area
- working effectively with others on the health care team
- staying within the bounds of your knowledge and skills
- providing safe care through understanding and following policies and procedures

Professional Conduct

Being a successful health care provider isn't just about remembering the facts you learned in school. It's about how you present yourself. The most knowledgeable person in the world will have trouble inspiring patients or coworkers with confidence if she seems rude, sarcastic, sloppy, or haphazard.

Remember that as a health care professional, every part of your personal conduct is scrutinized. Patients have to feel that they can trust you to take care of them. Your coworkers need to be reassured that you're capable of carrying out your responsibilities. You have to present yourself as a responsible person who is focused on work.

For a guideline, think back to doctors, nurses, and other health care providers you've come in contact with. How would you feel if they stood in the hall gossiping while you waited in the exam room? How would you feel if they seemed like they were rushing, irritated, or impatient? Health care demands a high standard of professional conduct from its members.

Go Team!

You might think of your clinical rotation as a time for you to shine by showing how much you've learned and what you can do. And it is. But it's also a time to show that you can be a successful member of a team.

Health care is all about teamwork. For example, an emergency medical technician takes critical vital signs and medical history before handing that information off to the doctor. The doctor makes evaluations based on this information and then orders lab work, x-rays, and medications. Every link in the chain is important. Even if you're in the front office or handling medical billing, your work is critically important to the members of the team providing direct care. By keeping patient records organized and up to date, you help ensure that the health care facility is able

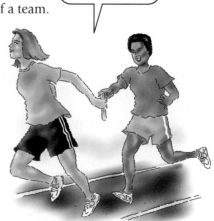

Every part of the team contributes to its success.

to provide the best care. Likewise, by sending the proper referrals and instructions to the lab, you enable lab personnel to perform necessary tests. And you can protect a patient's safety by informing the pharmacy of any
allergies the patient may have to certain drugs.

So, while you should take advantage of every opportunity to shine, remember that keeping the very complicated machinery of healthcare running is critically important. Being a reliable team member who can keep information flowing is very valuable.

Out of Bounds

Just as you have to be a team player to demonstrate professionalism, knowing the limits of your expertise makes you a trustworthy and professional health care provider.

There Are No Dumb Questions, Only Dumb Mistakes

There probably will be times when you think you know how to perform a certain task, but you're not completely sure. You may feel reluctant to ask for
verification—you might think it makes you look less than knowledgeable. You may be tempted to go with your hunch.

Stop! In health care, you have to be absolutely certain. If you have any questions about what you should do, ask someone who knows. Don't run the risk of making a mistake with a patient's records, medication, bloodwork, or other procedures. Instead, get the help you need and then carry out the task.

Know Your Limits

What if your supervisor or another staff person asks you to do something you haven't been trained to do? You might be very reluctant to admit that you don't know how to do the task. But it's a situation where you *must* say so. Remember, your clinical rotation is a learning experience. Everyone expects you to need guidance and training. No one expects you to know it all. The most important thing is that you stay within the bounds of your knowledge and skills.

Also, letting your supervisor and coworkers know your capabilities is vital to keeping the team running properly. Your team will trust you more if they know that you never attempt to do anything unless you're absolutely sure you know how to do it.

Read the Rule Book

In health care, it's important to do things by the book. Policies and procedures exist for every task, from filing to phlebotomy. And individual offices or departments may have additional rules that work well for them. These rules exist because if everyone in a facility does things the same way, there's never any confusion about what was done or how it was done.

One of the ways you can prepare for your clinical experience is to get a copy of the policy and procedures manual ahead of time so you can study it. Once you're on the job, know where the manual is stored and refer to it before trying a new procedure. When you're practicing at a facility, you must follow its procedures, even if you learned slightly different procedures at school.

Some of the policies and procedures may seem tedious. But you need to follow them to the letter every time. The biggest reason is safety. Following procedures means you won't have to worry about doing things incorrectly. If a patient develops a problem, you'll know that you didn't contribute to it. You can confidently report to your supervisors that you performed your tasks accurately. Also, you can one day train others to keep the team working smoothly and safely.

CONFIDENTIALITY

Only certain individuals can lawfully receive verbal, written, or electronic patient information. Those who have a need to know patient information include the patient's health care providers and those authorized by the patient to have access to that information. Private patient information includes things, such as:

- health records
- data on billing and payment
- insurance information
- prescriptions
- symptoms and diagnoses
- test results

Keeping Patient Information Private

You might overhear coworkers sharing patient information with each other in a casual way, over lunch or in the break room. If they encourage you to join in, remember that discussing private patient information is not only unprofessional, it's illegal. So, change the subject or just plead ignorance. If you never have information to share, others will soon stop asking you. This may be difficult, but it's better than getting yourself and your workplace into legal trouble for breaching patient privacy.

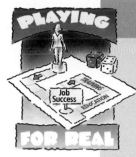

LIPS ZIPPED

Hi, I'm Donna and I'm training to become a home health aide. I was taking a break with some coworkers one day when they started talking about a couple of patients. They were saying things about the patients' homes and family situations that were very personal. Even though they weren't using the patients' names, I knew this kind of talk was inappropriate. They asked me if I'd been to one of the patient's homes and what I thought about it. I was tempted to get into it, but I knew it wasn't the right thing to do. So I just said, "I don't think we should be talking about this," and changed the subject by asking a question about a homework assignment.

The Health Insurance Portability and Accountability Act

The Health Insurance Portability and Accountability Act of 1996, or HIPAA, protects the privacy, confidentiality, and security of all medical records. During your clinical orientation, you'll receive information about maintaining patient rights under HIPAA. The information will be tailored to the health care facility where you're working. Failure to comply with HIPAA regulations, whether intentional or unintentional, can result in civil penalties. (See *Patient Privacy Rights.*)

Tips for Maintaining Patient Privacy

Some safeguards to help you maintain patient privacy include:

- protecting your computer password and logging off the computer when you're finished with it. Don't run the risk of an unauthorized person walking by and accessing patient information.

- keeping patient charts closed or put away when not in use.

- making sure faxes and computer printouts are not left unattended, especially in areas where curious patients are waiting, like the front desk.

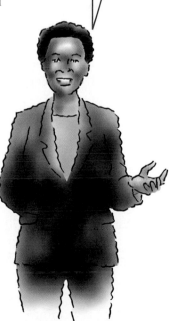

Never share a patient's personal information with anyone except those allowed under HIPAA rules.

- disposing of unneeded patient information in special receptacles before you leave the facility.

- keeping patient information out of your casual conversations. This means no conversation about patient information with patient visitors, or even with your family and friends.

- using a low voice when giving necessary information to others on the health care team, whether on the telephone or in person. A listening patient might spread details to other people.

- removing patient identifying information before handing in written class work.

PATIENT PRIVACY RIGHTS

The goal of HIPAA is to provide safeguards against inappropriate use and release of personal medical information, including all medical records and identifiable health information in any form (electronic, paper, and verbal). HIPAA gives patients the right to:

- give consent before information is released for treatments, payment, or health care operations.

- be educated about the provider's policy on privacy protection.

- access their health records.

- request that their health records be amended for accuracy.

- access the history of non-routine disclosures (disclosures that didn't occur in the course of treatment, payment, health care operations, or those not specifically authorized by the patient).

- request that the provider restrict the use and routine disclosure of information she has. (Providers aren't required to grant this request, especially if they think the information is important to the quality of patient care, such as disclosing HIV status to another medical treatment provider.)

PATIENT RIGHTS AND SAFETY

Concern for patients' rights and safety should be another part of your professional code of ethics. By keeping these things in mind, you'll not only protect your workplace from legal action, you'll also be providing the best care to patients.

The Right to Be Involved

Patients are more knowledgeable, assertive, and actively involved in their health care than ever before. They analyze their own symptoms and question their doctors' diagnoses. Some patients even perform home testing before visiting a health care facility. Patients also demand more education about the risks, alternatives, and benefits associated with the treatment recommended by their doctors. Bills of rights for patients have helped reinforce the public's expectation of quality care. (See *Patient's Bill of Rights*.)

As a member of the health care team, you need to uphold all patient rights as you carry out your duties. Become familiar with your employer's policy on patient rights. View your patients as partners in the health care process and help them get involved in their treatment and care.

PATIENT'S BILL OF RIGHTS

In 1977, the National League for Nursing (NLN) published a patient's bill of rights.

- People have the right to health care that's accessible and that meets professional standards, regardless of where they receive care.

- Patients have the right to courteous and individualized health care that is equitable, humane, and given without discrimination as to race, color, creed, sex, national origin, source of payment, or ethical or political beliefs.

- Patients have the right to information about their diagnosis, prognosis, and treatment, including alternatives to care and risks involved in care, in terms they and their families can easily understand, so they can give informed consent.

- Patients have the legal right to informed participation in all decisions concerning their health care.

- Patients have the right to information about the qualifications, names, and titles of personnel responsible for providing their health care.

- Patients have the right to refuse observation by those not directly involved in their care.

- Patients have the right to privacy during interview, exam, and treatment.

- Patients have the right to privacy in communicating and visiting with persons of their choice.

- Patients have the right to refuse treatments, medications, or participation in research and experimentation, without punitive action being taken against them.
- Patients have the right to coordination and continuity of health care.
- Patients have the right to appropriate instruction or education from health care personnel so they can achieve an optimal level of wellness and an understanding of their basic health needs.
- Patients have the right to confidentiality of all records (except as otherwise provided for by law or third-party payer contracts) and all communications, written or verbal, between patients and health care providers.
- Patients have the right of access to all health records pertaining to them, the right to challenge and to have their records corrected for accuracy, and the right to transfer all such records in the case of continuing care.
- Patients have the right to information on the charges for services, including the right to challenge these.
- Above all, patients have the right to be fully informed as to all their rights in all health care settings.

Reprinted with permission from the National League for Nursing. National League for Nursing. (1977). *Nursing's role in patients' rights*. New York: Author.

Keep Patients Safe!

Patient safety is the responsibility of all members of the health care team, including you. Even if you don't deal with patients in the exam room, you still need to focus on safety. Patient safety is your responsibility whether you see a patient in the front office or in the examination room.

Safety concerns will vary according to facility type and patient capability and needs. You can, however, take basic steps to reduce each patient's risk.

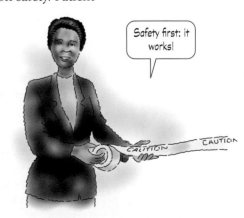

Safety first: it works!

Trip-and-Fall Hazards

Falls can be caused by many factors: medication, debris on the floor, or out-of-place equipment. So be vigilant and protective of your patients. Even if you feel that your work area is well out of range for patient falls, remember that patients travel through most parts of a facility. As the receptionist, for example, you might want to check the waiting area periodically to make sure there are no magazines on the ground, tables too close to chairs, or large potted plants too close to seats. All of these are potential trip-and-fall hazards.

Equipment Safety

You're responsible for making sure the equipment you have been trained and authorized to use for patient care is free from defects. You're also responsible for using that equipment properly and following instructions in the procedure manual. If you have questions about equipment use, ask your supervisor or instructor.

Decrease Disease

To reduce the risk of transmitting disease, wash your hands! Proper hand washing (with soap and water or water-less soap) is the single most effective thing you can do to prevent the spread of infection.

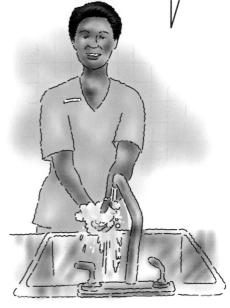

Wash your hands after procedures, even if you were wearing gloves.

Protect Yourself!

While providing safe care for patients, you also must protect yourself. Prevention is the key to keeping yourself safe in the workplace.

Infection: The Buck Stops Here

To protect yourself from infection, you should handle the following as if they contain infectious organisms:

- all blood and other body fluids
- human tissue
- mucous membranes
- broken skin

This means you should follow standard precautions at all times. For example, you must wear gloves for procedures that might expose you to a patient's blood or other body fluids. (See *Stop the Spread of Infection.*) Even if a patient appears healthy, the same precautions always apply.

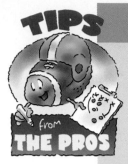

STOP THE SPREAD OF INFECTION

The Centers for Disease Control and Prevention (CDC) developed guidelines to provide the widest possible protection against the transmission of infection. CDC officials recommend that health care workers handle all blood and other body fluids, tissues, mucous membranes, and broken skin as if they contained infectious agents, regardless of the patient's diagnosis, and to take the following precautions.

• Wash your hands before and after patient care, after removing gloves, or immediately after contamination with blood, body fluids, excretions, secretions, or drainage.

• Wear gloves if you will or might come in contact with blood or other body fluids, specimens, tissues, secretions, excretions, mucous membranes, broken skin, or contaminated objects or surfaces.

• Change gloves and wash your hands between patients. When caring for the same patient, change gloves and wash your hands if you touch anything with a high concentration of microorganisms.

• Wear a fluid-resistant gown, eye protection, and a mask during procedures that are likely to generate droplets of blood or bodily fluids.

• Carefully handle used patient care equipment that's soiled with blood or body fluids; follow facility guidelines for cleaning and disinfecting equipment and environmental surfaces.

• Keep contaminated linens away from your body and place in properly labeled containers.

• Handle needles and sharps carefully and immediately discard in an impervious disposal unit after use; use sharps with safety features whenever possible.

• Immediately notify your supervisor of a needle-stick or sharp instrument injury, mucosal splash, or contamination of non-intact skin with blood or other body fluids to initiate appropriate investigation of the incident and care.

• Use mouthpieces, resuscitation bags, or ventilation devices in place of mouth-to-mouth resuscitation.

- Place a patient in a private room if he can't maintain hygiene measures or may contaminate the environment.
- If occupational exposure to blood is likely, you should be vaccinated against hepatitis B.
- Become familiar with your facility's infection control policies and procedures.

When Accidents Happen...

If you do receive an injury from a sharp instrument, or if any of your mucous membranes become contaminated by blood or other body fluids, notify your clinical instructor immediately. She will:

- help you with immediate first aid
- fill out an accident report
- ensure that you receive the proper follow-up care

Depending on your duties during your clinical rotation, you may be at risk of occupational exposure to hepatitis B. If so, your school might require you to get the hepatitis B vaccine series.

Be Kind to Your Back

Back injuries are common among health care employees. Many patient care facilities and laboratories require you to push, pull, lift, and carry heavy objects or equipment. People working in records or billing may have boxes of files to move. By using proper body mechanics, you can avoid back injuries.

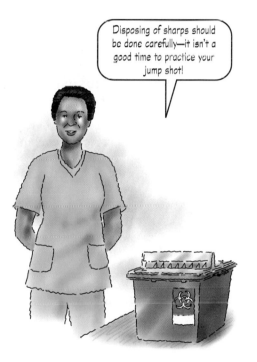

Disposing of sharps should be done carefully—it isn't a good time to practice your jump shot!

- Keep a low center of gravity by flexing your hips and knees instead of bending at the waist. This position distributes weight evenly between your upper and lower body and helps maintain balance.
- Create a wide base of support by spreading your feet apart. This tactic provides lateral stability and lowers your body's center of gravity.

- Maintain proper body alignment and keep your body's center of gravity directly over the base of support by moving your feet rather than twisting and bending at the waist.

Handle Chemicals With Care

Many potentially hazardous chemicals are used in health care facilities. Certain drugs, powerful cleaning solutions, and disinfectants are common hazards. A material safety data sheet (MSDS) provides you with information about the physical and chemical hazards that can occur from these substances. Each MSDS provides information about the chemicals found in a substance and how to treat exposure to that substance. Each health care facility will have an MSDS manual. Make sure you know where the manual is located in your facility.

CULTURAL DIVERSITY

Your clinical experience will probably bring you into contact with a wide variety of people, including patients, doctors, and other staff members from culturally diverse backgrounds. When people talk about cultural diversity, they are referring to the ways in which all people are similar to and different from each other. Racial classifications, ethnicity, gender, sexual orientation, religious affiliation, socioeconomic status, and age are all elements of cultural diversity.

It's natural to note differences between yourself and those around you. Regardless of these differences, part of your professional code as a health care provider demands that you treat everyone with equal care and respect. This means refusing to allow any preconceived notions you may have about others to affect the quality of your work. By recognizing that we all make judgments about people, we can move closer toward appreciating the things that make people different and treating everyone with the same care and respect.

Cultural diversity is an important part of health care because of the genetic characteristics, cultural values, and belief systems that affect people's health. By knowing and understanding these cultural differences, you'll be able to provide better care.

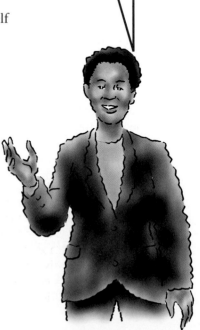

Part of being a professional means treating everyone you encounter—patients, supervisors, and coworkers—with equal care and respect.

Race and Ethnicity

The term *race* is typically based on a person's physical characteristics, such as skin color, facial features, hair texture, and body stature. *Ethnicity* is the concept of identifying with the traditions and values of a particular cultural group. Although the terms ethnicity and race are often used interchangeably, they refer to different aspects of a person's identity. An individual can be of one race, yet identify with a different ethnicity.

Race is sometimes a factor in diagnosis and treatment because genetic traits are often more common in certain racial groups than in others. Likewise, ethnic values and traditions also can have an effect on a patient's health and well-being.

Gender Roles

It's important to consider gender roles when working with patients. In some cultures, the male is considered the head of the household. In these cases, a male family member might speak for his female family members. In other cultures, women are the dominant family members. It's important that health care professionals consider this when providing care. Gender roles may influence the way in which a patient prefers to be treated. Every patient has a different role in the family, and it's important to be sensitive to the different needs and priorities of each.

Sexual Orientation

A patient's sexual orientation is often a personal matter. A patient may choose whether or not to discuss her sexual orientation with her health care provider. There are times, however, when sexual orientation may be an important issue (for example, in addressing sexually transmitted diseases). Regardless of what information patients choose to reveal, it's important to avoid making judgments or assumptions about a patient's sexual orientation or lifestyle choices.

Religion

Patients' religious beliefs and values may affect the way in which they wish to be treated by health care professionals. For example, a person's religious affiliation can influence his decisions concerning diet and nutrition, sexual lifestyle, and other health matters. As a health care professional, you'll need to be sensitive to each patient's values and beliefs when providing care. You can do this by respecting the personal choices made by patients and adapting care to suit each patient's needs.

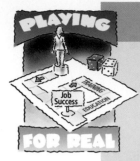

KEEPING AN OPEN MIND

My name is Ling, and I'm a medical assistant. There was one patient I came across during my clinical experience who I thought had something against women. He wouldn't let me take his blood pressure—he always asked for a man to do it. I thought he was prejudiced against me, so I talked to my mentor about it. She told me that I shouldn't make assumptions or take his actions personally. She said that part of providing the best care meant doing what I could to accommodate different patients' needs, whether they make sense to me or not.

Later, I found out that the patient is an Orthodox Jew, and it's against his religion to be touched by a woman who's not in his family. I was embarrassed about my assumptions. After that, I made sure a male medical assistant was around to take the patient's blood pressure and other vital signs during his office visits.

Socioeconomic Status

A person's socioeconomic status should not affect the kind of care and treatment that a health care professional provides. Every patient, regardless of financial situation, should be given the best possible care and attention. Put patients' social or economic standing out of your mind while you're providing care. Avoid stereotyping patients according to their level of education or how much money they make. Instead, focus on each patient as an individual worthy of your attention, respect, and sensitivity.

Age

The aging process will affect the health of every patient in different ways. Younger patients will have different health care needs than older patients. You'll need to be sensitive to patients' changing physical and emotional needs as they grow older. It's also essential that you avoid making assumptions about a patient based on age. It is important to remember that physical fitness and health can vary for different people at every age and stage in their lives.

PERSONAL CONDUCT

When you work in health care, your personal conduct really matters. Patients will probably see you face to face, whether you're providing direct care or taking their insurance information. They'll size up your character and make decisions about whether they can trust you and whether you seem to care about them.

Patients also give you information that is very private—sometimes information not even their families know about. So you have to be the kind of person a patient can trust. There are three main characteristics you need to have to be a good health care professional:

- *Integrity.* Be recognized as someone with good character.
- *Dependability.* Be someone who always does what she's supposed to do.
- *Trustworthiness.* Be someone who consistently does the right thing and is always honest.

Integrity

Integrity refers to the quality of your character. As you learned in Chapter 3, the character you develop as a student will influence the character you'll have as a health care professional. That's why it's important to start thinking about your character now, while you're in school.

Someone with integrity stands by her personal code of ethics. She's honest in everything she does and accepts accountability for her actions. This quality is especially important to have as a health care professional. Someone with integrity will be sure to keep patient information private and will be honest about her actions—even when she makes mistakes.

Dependability

Dependability is crucial in health care. Medical facilities are busy places, which makes teamwork necessary to everyday office operations. Even one person not showing up to work or coming late can throw off the entire day. As a member of the health care team, you need to be there—your teammates are counting on you! Be someone who always makes it in to work on time.

Dependability also applies to the quality of your work. If you're asked to perform a task, you should always perform it when you are told to and

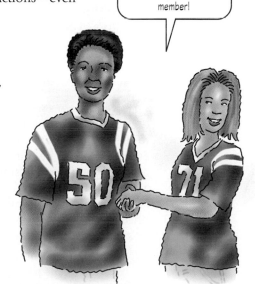

In health care, you have to be a dependable team member!

to the exact specifications you are given. In the hectic world of the health care facility, delays and mistakes add up to late hours and unhappy patients.

Being dependable means that you'll always follow through and do what you're asked. It means that your coworkers, supervisors, and patients can feel comfortable putting their trust in you and relying on you to get the job done.

Trustworthiness

Being trustworthy means people can feel confident knowing you can be trusted in all situations and that you'll always do the right thing. Even as a health care professional, you may be tempted to cut corners or do things that are not quite on the up and up. Being trustworthy means you stand firm in your commitment to honesty, forthrightness, and doing things the right way. Not only will you feel good about yourself when you're trustworthy, but you'll also earn and keep the respect of everyone around you.

Planning Ahead

As you look forward to your upcoming clinical rotation, there are some ways you can prepare for it so you hit the ground running on your first day.

- Know the dress code.
- Know the equipment.
- Know your mentor.
- Know the clinic.

SUIT UP

Professionalism starts with something that might seem trivial: dress. Just as athletes have to suit up before a game, you'll need to dress appropriately for *your* big game—your clinical experience. You might be thinking that just wearing your uniform protects you from dressing incorrectly. Not true! Yes, you probably will be wearing a uniform (for example, scrubs). But there are still important points to keep in mind to make sure you're dressed appropriately.

- Keep your uniform clean. This can be hard to do in a clinical setting, but it's important. A stained or wrinkled uniform tells patients and staff members that you don't take your work seriously.

- Wear your identification badge pinned near your collarbone. Clipping it to the bottom hem of your shirt makes it less visible to people who need to see who you are.

- Choose professional shoes. This usually means white shoes. Don't wear sneakers, sandals, or clogs unless you know for sure that they're allowed where you'll be working.

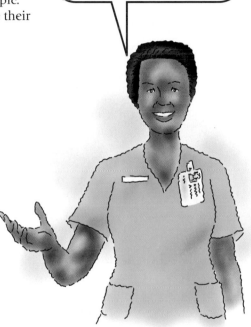

"Suiting up" for your clinical rotation means dressing like a true health care professional. Check with your clinical mentor if you have any questions about dress.

Aside from your uniform, there is another dress factor to keep in mind: keep it simple. Many people are tempted to personalize their uniforms with jewelry, perfume or cologne, or an unusual hairstyle. But when you're at work, you shouldn't stand out because of your original look. You should stand out because of your excellent skills and positive attitude. Professionals don't call attention to their looks on the job. They let their skills do the talking.

Some health care facilities have stricter guidelines about dress than others. Ask any questions you may have about dress code during your clinical orientation. Your clinical mentor or instructor will be able to provide you with specific guidelines to follow. If you're ever unsure as to whether a particular item of clothing or accessory is appropriate, play it safe until you've checked with your instructor.

KNOW THE EQUIPMENT

Your school will provide you with a list of equipment you'll need for your clinical rotation. Make sure you have all necessary supplies with you on your first day. You should also bring:

- a notebook
- a pen or pencil
- your personal identification (such as a Social Security card, driver's license, or an identification card issued by your school)

These additional items will come in handy in case you need to fill out any paperwork on your first day. You also might need proof of identification to obtain a parking permit or an identification badge. If you plan on driving to the facility every day, write down your car's license plate number in your notebook; you might need to register your car with the facility if you'll be parking in a garage.

Another helpful piece of equipment is a personal data assistant (PDA). Software for a PDA can take the place of a drug book, textbook, and other references. PDAs, as well as many cell phones, also have functions that can simplify your life, such as a calculator, address book, calendar, to-do list, and memo pad.

KNOW YOUR MENTOR

Your clinical mentor (or preceptor) will coach you through your clinical experience. Do your best to start out on the right foot with your mentor—you just might learn something! Also, try to avoid making unfair judgments about your mentor based on what you may have heard from other students. Get to know your mentor before forming an opinion.

No Name Games

Remember to be polite and respectful. Address your mentor as Mr., Mrs., Dr., Ms., or by a first name, according to your mentor's stated preference. It's part of the mutual respect you want in your relationship.

Background Check

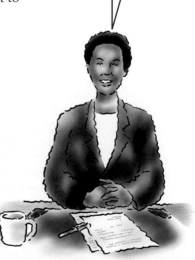

Work with your mentor to make your clinical rotation a positive experience.

Try to learn a little bit about how your mentor arrived at where he is today. For instance, you could ask questions about how he got into health care, where he went to school, and the positions he has held. You don't have to pry or overwhelm him with questions. These topics are general enough to come up in conversation.

You should have regular conversations with your mentor about what you're learning and doing. You don't have to worry that this will impose on him. He'll be happy to answer your questions and to see that you're eager to learn.

Head off Trouble

If you feel you're unable to develop a good relationship with your mentor, make an appointment to discuss your concerns. If you can't resolve the problems together, follow the procedures outlined in your student handbook for resolving grievances.

KNOW THE FACILITY

Every health care facility has some unique procedures. Learn how your particular facility does things so you can fit in with the team as soon as possible. Two important steps to learning the ropes are:

1. Attend your clinical orientation.
2. Work out the logistics before your first day.

Clinical Orientation

Clinical orientation usually takes place at the facility where you'll be doing your rotation. It typically includes a welcome from a representative of the facility, followed by information about the facility's:

- mission statement
- fire and safety procedures
- confidentiality rules

If you need computer access, your orientation may also include computer classes and password assignment.

Your mentor will explain her expectations for your rotation. She'll give you a schedule to follow, and she'll explain written assignments and due dates. Clinical objectives and evaluation procedures also will be reviewed at this time, so be sure to ask questions if you have them.

Logistics

There are a lot of smaller details you'll need to consider before you begin your clinical experience. Where should you park? Whom do you call if you're going to be late or out sick? Do you need to wear a pager when you leave the facility for lunch?

Remember to ask these types of questions during orientation. The last thing you want at the end of your first day is to find that your car has been towed. Or, if you don't know whom to notify if you're going to be late or absent, that information could be passed along

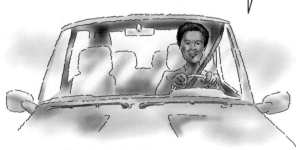

Make sure you get to work on time—take traffic and parking into consideration.

to several people before it gets to the one person who needs it. And you don't want to come back from lunch to find out that everyone has been frantically looking for you!

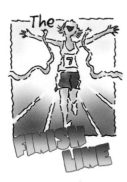

- Protect patient rights by familiarizing yourself with the Patient's Bill of Rights.
- Guard patient privacy by following HIPAA rules.
- Learn about your facility's safety rules by reading the policy and procedures manual.
- Develop a code of ethics. Bring qualities, such as integrity, dependability, and trustworthiness, into your career as a health care professional.
- Plan for a successful clinical experience. Dress appropriately, bring the right books and supplies, and make sure you arrive on time!

Review Questions

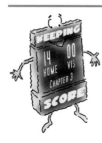

1. How can you practice skills in a clinical setting before your rotation begins?
2. Why is it important to know your limits when you're working in health care?
3. Describe your mentor's role in your clinical experience.

Chapter Activities

1. Calm Your Fears: Review the chapter. Make a list of the aspects of your upcoming clinical experience that cause you the most anxiety. Come up with concrete questions to ask your instructor about each troubling aspect. Put your most urgent question at the top and work your way down the list.

2. Act It Out: Get together with three to five classmates. Have each person write down a clinical procedure she is nervous about performing. Then act out each procedure with the group, first with other members showing how the procedure is done, then letting the person who was nervous try it by herself.

Chapter 9

YOUR FUTURE SUCCESS

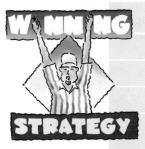

- See your dreams becoming reality

- Understand the positive choices you make each day

- Recognize the obstacles you've overcome

- Take pride in the goals you've met

- Explain how to carry your new skills and knowledge into the future

Now that you're nearing the end of this book, it's a good time to look back on what brought you to this point. Are you closer to fulfilling your original dreams? What obstacles have you overcome along the way? What goals have you accomplished? What skills and knowledge will you be able to use in the future?

Remembering Where You Started

You've come a long way since you first opened this book. You've learned how to:

- set and meet goals
- plan ahead and be prepared
- schedule multiple activities and meet deadlines
- identify and deal with stress and anxiety
- listen effectively and apply your critical thinking skills
- meet the challenges of learning and take responsibility for the results
- network and contribute in group activities

- explore optional resources to help you get ahead
- meet standards of professionalism and uphold patients' rights

Why is it important to see how far you've come? Because thinking about your successes can be an encouragement and a great way to find the motivation you need to tackle the next challenge!

Imagine yourself 5 or 10 years down the road. Now look at the list above of all of the things that you have already learned. You can apply every one of these new skills to help you succeed in all of your future career and education goals. Ask any health-care professional and they'll readily agree, for example, that being able to schedule multiple activities and plan ahead are critical to their job success.

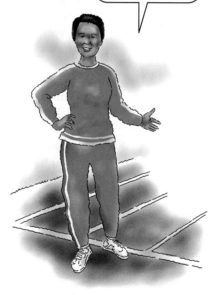

Now it's time to look back on just how far you've come.

You see, it isn't just about getting through this book, or this class. You've paved the way to much, much more! So let's take a look at the dreams you have for your future, the courage you've shown in facing your fears about school, and the wise choices you've made so far.

DREAMS

When you started school with your eye on a new career, you may have dreamed of improving your lifestyle, supporting your family, or gaining self-respect. Whichever dream got you started, you are now much closer to making that dream a reality.

Even if you're still a few years away from starting your career in health care, you have done the hardest, most important part: taking action. You tackled the sometimes difficult and complicated task of applying to school and enrolling in courses. You shuffled your work and other responsibilities to make time for class. You studied hard and completed your coursework. All these things have brought you closer to making your dream a reality.

Down the road a few years, after you've been in your new healthcare role for a while, you may begin to think you are ready for another challenge. Perhaps you will start out as a Medical Assistant, but you start dreaming of being the Clinic Manager. Or maybe you will finish your Radiology Technician program, and decide that you really like caring for cancer patients, so you dream of specializing in oncology radiology.

It's great to have new dreams and aspirations. The experiences you've had so far in making your dreams a reality will help you take on new challenges and new dreams in the future.

Therefore, it's important to recognize and take pride in your accomplishments, no matter how small they may seem at the time. Celebrate each success now, whether it's doing well on a test, completing a research project, or forming a study group with a few fellow students. Remember, it's the small steps that move you toward accomplishing big things!

COURAGE

How did you face your fears about school and learning? You had courage! It's very hard to embrace the unknown. You may have been nervous about continuing your education. Maybe you also had to face grumbling about your new schedule from coworkers, supervisors, or family members. Proving that you can live up to your old responsibilities while taking on new ones takes courage, too!

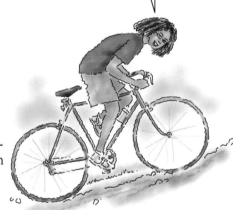

I *can* do this, and it *is* worth it!

Picture once again where you'll be 5 or 10 years down the road. Right now it may be hard to imagine that you'll actually be the Clinic Manager, or the cancer center's Oncology Radiology Technician. But it's possible! You've shown to yourself and proved to those around you that you have the courage and fortitude to stick with it and meet your goals. It takes courage to believe in yourself and to believe that you can make changes in terms of your education and future career. It takes courage to say, "I *can* do this, and it *is* worth it."

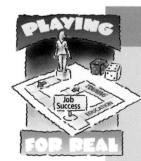

HAVING THE COURAGE TO SUCCEED

My name is Leila. When I first thought about starting school, I was intimidated. It was a big financial and emotional investment for my family and me. What if I couldn't handle it and had to drop out after one semester? I was worried about what people would think. But then I remembered how my uncle always used to say, "Nothing ventured, nothing gained." If I never took a chance, I'd never achieve anything. I decided it was better to take a chance than to tell myself I couldn't do it.

CHOICES

To make it this far, you had to have faith in your choices. You've had to make decisions about:

- which school to attend
- what courses to take
- which degree or certificate plan to pursue

Those were your biggest choices. Some of your smaller, but important decisions may have been sticking to your study schedule rather than "winging it," or initiating a study group rather than going it alone, or implementing some stress relief techniques instead of suffering. Every day, you make small decisions that keep your dream of success alive.

You'll need to continue to make both big and small choices as you continue on your career path. For example, there may be some small aspect of your job that you don't love—maybe you find getting the surgical instruments ready for sterilizing to be a little tedious, even though you *love* the biggest part of your job—assisting the surgical team when they are performing operations on patients.

Do you give up being a Surgical Technician altogether because of one small aspect you don't enjoy? Probably not. Professional hockey players may not like getting up before dawn to hit the ice for practice, but they do it because the payoff—playing the game they love at the highest level—is worth it. You can do the same in your job. You will discover ways to make small sacrifices in order to live your dream. Who knows, one day you may be the head surgical tech, and cleaning instruments will no longer be a part of your job!

Obstacles You Overcame Along the Way

You know it hasn't been easy to arrive at where you are today. You have overcome many obstacles already. Throughout this book, you have learned how to:

- keep a positive attitude
- shake off fear, doubt, and discouragement
- stay motivated
- manage stress
- handle work and personal life conflicts

How have you overcome these obstacles to your success? For example, if others discouraged you in the beginning, perhaps you overcame that obstacle by surrounding yourself with more supportive people. If you doubted your abilities as a student, you may have gained confidence with each new positive experience at school.

In life, everyone faces challenges. In your future career you will *definitely* face new challenges. For example, we all know that things change, and nothing is changing faster than the healthcare field! So your job will undoubtedly also change. You will be given new responsibilities and you'll be asked to do more. As technology advances, you'll be expected to learn new skills and ride the wave of progress. Those who can rise to meet these new challenges become successful. Remember that the obstacles you face are not as important as how you choose to handle them!

> Touchdown! Every time you overcome an obstacle to your success, take time to celebrate!

ATTITUDE: KEEP IT POSITIVE!

The key to success is often inside your own head. If you believe you can do something, you'll find a way to do it. Believing in yourself—having a positive attitude—is the first step toward accomplishing your goals. A positive attitude helps you identify and accept your responsibilities in the learning process and on the job. It also helps you set performance goals for yourself. This has already helped you study effectively and continually improve your grades. Five or 10 years from now, your positive attitude will continue to help you advance in your career.

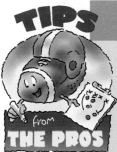

SHAKE IT OFF!

When you get nervous about the obstacles you face, you can become fearful of them. This leads you to doubt your ability to overcome those obstacles, which might make you discouraged. Taking small steps can help you shake off those feelings of fear, doubt, and discouragement.

For example, one of the biggest challenges you may have faced is learning how to be an active learner. When you're working and going to class, as well as fulfilling other responsibilities, you may not have a lot of energy left to ask questions in class, visit your instructor during office hours, join a study group, take on an internship, or go the extra mile to get your education.

But as you took each of these small steps, it probably became easier to extend yourself. Now that you're in the habit of being an active learner, it's become second nature. And there are other things you can do to become an even more active learner. If you joined a study group, why not lead one? If you know what field you want to enter, why not set up some informational interviews with professionals working in that field? It's just a matter of taking what you're already doing one step further.

And being an active learner now is good practice for being a go-getter on the job. Everyone knows that the go-getters do better in their chosen careers. Think about it. If you had to hire someone to get things done, would you choose the applicant who waited to be told what to do?

FINDING YOUR MOTIVATION

When you have a positive attitude, it's easier to stay motivated. School takes effort. If you're motivated to make the necessary effort, you'll be able to stay on track with your school and career goals.

You can find motivation by reflecting on your past successes, big and small. Whether it's doing well on your final exam or just getting through a very busy day, focusing on your achievements can help you stay motivated for the tasks ahead.

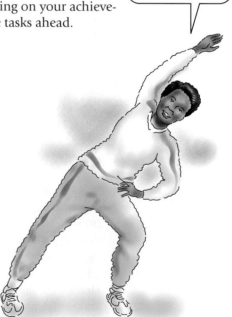

Stretch yourself to become an even more active learner!

Sources of Motivation

As you learned in Chapter 1, you might be motivated intrinsically (within yourself) or extrinsically (by outside benefits)—or even a combination of both. As you've read this book, you've probably discovered various ways to motivate yourself in school. Remember, you can find motivation inside yourself by calling on:

- your desires to learn and do well
- your curiosity about new subjects and new skills
- your sense of adventure in being willing to take risks

If those things don't inspire you, try

seeking out extrinsic motivation instead, such as:

- improved grades and higher GPA
- better self-esteem and the esteem of your colleagues
- accomplishments you can add to your resume
- a better job with a higher salary

Where have you found motivation? What—and who—has helped you stay motivated? Take a moment to write down a few challenges you have faced and what motivated you to face them.

Motivation Bonuses

When you motivate yourself to succeed in school, you do well in other areas of your life, too. You become a more successful person. The skills required to do well in school apply to all life challenges:

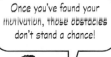

Once you've found your motivation, those obstacles don't stand a chance!

- *Persistence.* Learning how to keep doing your best even during difficult times is a very important life skill. In health care, there are difficult times. For example, during cold and flu season, demands on your time at work will be greater and your work days more hectic. Everyone has tough times; it's how you respond to them that matters.

- *Confidence.* It takes confidence to approach an instructor and ask for help or extra information. Later, your confidence may help you to approach your supervisor with a new idea, to ask for a raise, or to change a schedule. You'll also need confidence in dealing with difficult patients.

- *Networking.* At school, other students can be valuable sources of information and support. At work, coworkers can offer the same benefits. Networking also teaches you how to offer value to those around you. Before you know it, you may find others trying to network with you!

- *Focus.* Working through distractions is an invaluable skill, whether you're in class or in the middle of a task at work. Healthcare is a very busy business! Your ability to focus and stay on task will be put to the test daily.

- *Self-discipline.* No one can do your work for you. It sounds simple, but many people never learn this. Being self-disciplined means you are the kind of "self-starter" all employers are looking for.
- *Planning.* In school, you have to plan for study time, class time, tests, and so much more to accomplish everything. At work, you'll need to create a schedule that allows you to get everything done efficiently and accurately.
- *Keeping a positive outlook.* You have to believe that what you're doing is worthwhile and that you have what it takes to succeed. With this attitude, you won't dwell on setbacks or spread negative rumors. Everyone enjoys working with a person who is a pleasure to be around!

When you're able to deal with all aspects of your life in the same confident and motivated way, you'll find yourself better able to deal with challenges.

ON THE OFFENSE AGAINST STRESS

You've learned a lot about managing stress. It may not seem like it, but there are probably several stressors you've shaken off by now:

- wondering what school will be like
- wondering if you'll be able to keep up with your new schedule
- wondering if you can succeed as a student

When going up against the stresses of your career, remember to use some of the offensive moves you've learned as a student, such as:

- setting priorities
- simplifying your day-to-day life
- learning how to say no occasionally
- keeping your mind and body healthy

Set Priorities

Setting priorities means determining which commitments are necessary and which commitments or tasks aren't. As you look at each task on your daily to-do list, ask yourself, "Is it absolutely necessary to get this task done today, or would it just be *nice* to get it done today?" Move the absolutely necessary tasks to the top of your list. After—and only after—those tasks have been accomplished, consider tackling the other items. If you're unable to complete all the tasks on your list, don't stress. Instead, feel good about everything you did manage to accomplish that day.

If some activities are constantly falling toward the bottom of your list, you might need to cut those activities out of your schedule entirely. You may not have time for everything, but by setting priorities, you can make time for the most important things.

Keep It Simple

One strategy for avoiding stress on the job as well as in your daily life is to simplify. It helps to get organized. For example, if you can complete several errands or tasks in one trip because they all take you to the same place, you can check a few things off your to-do list at once. Avoid participating in optional activities if they take up valuable time. At work, this might be chatting with your coworkers. Learn to say no when you have too much to do. Also, remember to take time for relaxing when the job's done!

Healthy Body, Healthy Mind

A fit and well-rested body can withstand stress better than a tired and run-down body. Remember to exercise for 30 minutes at least three times a week. Many working people exercise during their lunch break. Exercise may seem like a luxury, but it's a necessity for fighting stress. If you take good care of your body, you'll be better able to keep up with your busy schedule without becoming too stressed.

Food for Thought

Your brain needs nutrition to function properly. Eating right can give you the strength you'll need to be on the offensive against stress. You learned in Chapter 1 that vitamin B, vitamin C, and folic acid all help your body handle stress. You can get these nutrients from citrus fruits and leafy green vegetables.

Part of healthy eating also means having a balanced diet of vegetables, fruits, grains, and low-fat proteins. It's important to cut back on things like sugar, salt, saturated fat, and caffeine. Several cups of coffee each morning may seem like the best way to wake up and get moving, but caffeine can cause tension and anxiety. As a result, you may find it harder to deal with stress. If you're looking for an energy boost, it's best to rely on healthier options, such as eating nutritious foods, exercising regularly, and getting enough rest.

Sleep: How Much Is Enough?

When you're tired, you're more likely to feel helpless, incapable, and defeated. Nothing sabotages a positive attitude like fatigue. Make sure you get 8 hours of sleep each night. That may seem like a lot—another luxury—but it's necessary for your emotional, mental, and physical health. Sleep is key to good performance in school, at work, and in life in general. By taking courses, you've been asking yourself to do more each day, so it's a good idea to give your body the rest it needs. And getting enough rest will help you do more in your job and make more of your career.

Relax Inside and Out

When you're stressed, your body reacts as if it's being attacked. Both your brain and the rest of your nervous system tense up. You can help back off from this "red alert" by relaxing your body and your mind.

For your body, try relaxation and stress management techniques, such as massage, yoga, and meditation. Exercise is another relaxation technique. When you're sweating on a treadmill, or pushing up a hill on your bike, exercise may not seem so relaxing. But after you finish your exercise session, you'll feel stronger, calmer, and more positive.

For your mind, focus on the positive. Try not to dwell on the stress you're facing. Acknowledge it and then move on to a solution. For example, you could start by acknowledging to yourself or a close friend that you're stressed about an upcoming test or the piles of paperwork waiting for you at work. Then, you could move on to a solution by making time to study thoroughly or by setting aside lower-priority tasks. It's also important to spend time with people who can help reinforce your positive thinking. Family, friends, classmates, and others can help you stay positive and remind you that people care about you no matter what. Other positive coworkers can remind you that you're all in this together.

Go-o-o-al!

When you think of your main goal as a student, you probably see yourself working in your new health care career. But you know there are many smaller goals between that future and the present:

- doing well in your courses
- learning new skills
- finding the right job

These are big-picture goals you'll reach by achieving smaller goals, such as keeping your study schedule, attending class, balancing work and school, and registering for the right courses.

Adjust your short-term goals to make sure you reach your long-term go-o-o-al!

YOUR GOALS AND YOU: A LONG-TERM RELATIONSHIP

You've already learned that your goals fall into these categories:

- *Long-term*. These are things you hope to accomplish in the next 5 to 10 years.
- *Intermediate*. These are things you would like to accomplish in the next 3 to 5 years.
- *Short-term*. These goals are 6 months to 2 years in the future.
- *Immediate*. These are things you hope to accomplish today, this week, or this month.

As you know, all of your goals need to be measurable, reachable, and desirable. Otherwise, you won't be motivated to reach them!

HOW ARE YOU DOING?

Take some time to evaluate your progress so far by writing your goals here.

Long-Term Goal (to be accomplished in the next 5 to 10 years):

1. _____

Intermediate Goals (to be accomplished in the next 3 to 5 years):

1. _____
2. _____

Short-Term Goals (to be accomplished in the next 6 months to 2 years):

1. _____
2. _____
3. _____

Immediate Goals (to be accomplished today, this week, or this month):

1. _____
2. _____
3. _____
4. _____
5. _____

Now, ask yourself these questions.

1. When I first started reading this book, what immediate or short-term goals had I hoped to accomplish by now? Have I accomplished these goals?

2. If there are goals I have not accomplished, what stopped me?

3. How did I accomplish my other goals?

4. What can I do differently next semester to make sure I meet all my immediate or short-term goals?

5. What are two or three new immediate goals I can accomplish today, this week, or this month?

CHANGE CAN BE GOOD

Students adjust their goals for many reasons. Maybe their original goals were proven to be unrealistic once they actually started school. Maybe as they began taking courses, they developed an interest in a slightly different career. These are good reasons to adjust your goals. If your original goals were unrealistic, there is no need to be embarrassed or frustrated. Being able to evaluate your original goals and make necessary changes is part of being a successful student. As you review your goals, ask yourself the following questions.

- Have any of my goals changed since I started school? If so, how and why have they changed?

- How do I feel when I make adjustments to my goals? Is it discouraging (I feel like I failed to meet my original goals) or empowering (I know I can adjust my goals without giving up on them)?

Remember, it's always better to modify your goals or your timeline than to give up!

When you make the decision to adjust your goals, keep in mind that the playing field is always changing. Once you become comfortable in one course, you move on to new courses with different instructors. After meeting one semester's scheduling challenges, you are soon met with a new set of scheduling challenges. Each of these situations can give you good reasons to adjust your goals, so try to avoid seeing your adjustments as failures. Instead, focus on finding creative ways to overcome obstacles and keep moving forward. Being flexible is critical to your success.

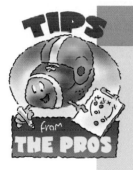

ADJUSTING YOUR GOALS

If you feel uncertain about your motives for adjusting your goals, talk to an academic advisor or someone else you trust.

1. Tell your advisor that you're thinking of making adjustments to your goals.
2. List the adjustments you're considering.
3. Give your reasons for considering the adjustments.
4. Ask your advisor if your reasons and adjustments seem positive or ask if there's a way you could meet your original goals.

If you talk to someone who is encouraging and supportive, you can feel at ease listening to that person's advice. But in the end, only you can decide if you really need to make changes to your goals.

A REWARDING EXPERIENCE

You may think of your graduation day as the time when you'll be rewarded for your hard work. Or maybe you picture the first day of your new career as your reward. But those long-term benefits may seem far away right now.

That's why you need to give yourself small rewards along the way. If you do well on a big test, for example, maybe you could go out with friends to celebrate. If you finish a big project you've been working on for weeks, consider taking a Saturday off to do something fun. If your study group has been working really hard, you could opt to meet at a local coffee shop once in a while for a more laid-back study session.

Promising yourself a reward at the end of a task can help motivate you to perform that task well. The kinds of rewards are up to you. The point is to reward yourself for all of your achievements, big and small, so you can stay motivated to keep going!

Carrying Your New Skills Into the Future

You're on the track to success as a student and in your career. You've learned a lot about what it takes to do well in school. Although your academic career may be just beginning, you already have:

- new skills and knowledge
- confidence and pride
- career focus

Five or 10 years from now, these things will be just as important.

SPEAKING THE LANGUAGE

You may feel like a rookie in your first semester or term at school, but you already know much more than you did before. You've begun to "speak the language" by picking up new knowledge and skills related to your future career. While your education may not be finished yet, partial knowledge is a big step up from no knowledge at all. And remember, learning is a lifelong process, especially in health care! Even as a professional, you'll continue to gain more knowledge and learn new techniques. The good learning habits you're developing now will continue to be useful for years to come.

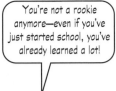

You're not a rookie anymore—even if you've just started school, you've already learned a lot!

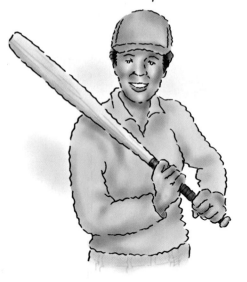

KNOWING YOUR WAY AROUND

In school, you're doing more than simply reading textbooks and going to class. You might be networking with your classmates, learning how to manage a busy new schedule, or making the most of all the campus resources available to students. Aside from being valuable experiences, these accomplishments can give you a sense of confidence and pride in your abilities. So, not only will you be able to bring useful skills into the workplace, you'll also have the confidence you'll need to get the job done!

The Networking Mogul

Right now, you're talking and working with fellow students— your future coworkers. You're making connections that might be helpful once you've entered your chosen career. And you're becoming a contact for others who respect your knowledge and your character.

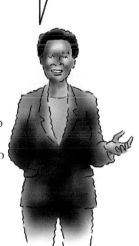

Learning the ropes will help you become more confident. And when you're working in health care, it's very important to be confident in your abilities!

The Scheduling Specialist

As a student, you're also getting to know the instructors and the types of courses they offer. You've learned about the different types of tests you'll face and how to prepare for them. Maybe you've also become a master scheduler. Learning to maintain your schedule through disruptions is a sign of success.

The Local Expert

Perhaps you're becoming an expert about your school. You know where all the offices and buildings are, you know whom to talk to for various problems, and you know how to use the library and its reference materials. It may be stressful to face obstacles as a student, but now you know where to go to get the help you need. And becoming an expert at school will make it easier to become an expert in the workplace. You'll be ahead of the game when it's easy for you to learn where everything is kept, who can help you solve problems, and how to get information quickly.

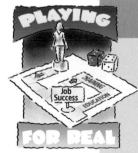

LEARNING THE ROPES

I'm Charles. When I first started school, I was really lost. The campus seemed huge. Every time I needed to do something, like sign up for courses or ask about my financial aid, I was told to go to some building I'd never heard of. My instructors all had materials on reserve at the library and I wasn't sure how to get them. And I was embarrassed to ask questions all the time. I thought it made me look dumb.

But there was no way around it, so I had to swallow my pride and ask. And you know what? I found out that people were happy to help me. No one thought I was dumb. After a few weeks, I didn't have the same problems any more—I knew where things were. Then *I* could be the one to help other students, which made me feel confident—like a leader. I realized that finding my way around campus wasn't an impossible challenge; it was just part of the learning process.

KNOWING WHAT TO EXPECT

Most importantly, you're learning more about the career you've chosen. Knowing what to expect helps you make informed decisions for your future.

Without knowing what's ahead, it's harder to plan and easier to become discouraged. You're in a better position now than before you started school. Now, you're aware of what lies ahead and you're prepared to face challenges that might otherwise have caused you to give up. Keep reminding yourself that you've come a long way so far; you owe it to yourself to keep going!

Getting Your First Professional Job

Soon you'll be looking for your first full-time job in health care, or a part-time or summer job for experience. You'll need a well-written résumé, an eye-catching cover letter, and polished interviewing skills. But where do you begin? Just as when you started school, the first step is the hardest. Here are some pointers to get you to the next step.

WRITING THE RÉSUMÉ

One thing to keep in mind about résumés is that they don't all have to follow the same format. A second thing to keep in mind is that one potential employer will like one type of résumé and another potential employer will like another type. What this means is that there is no one correct way to write a résumé. There are many Web sites that will help you. In fact, you can post your résumé directly onto some Web sites that conduct job searches. In any case, every résumé should include the basics:

- contact information—your name, phone number(s), address, and e-mail address
- education—relevant courses you've completed, diplomas, certifications or degrees you've earned, along with educational honors and achievements
- work experience—relevant positions you have held, along with your responsibilities and achievements in them, and the names and addresses of your past employers and the dates you worked for them

In addition, you should consider including

- your objective—the title of the job position you want, or one or two sentences about what you want to do

- skills, traits, and achievements relevant to the job—for example, computer skills, language skills, people skills, technical skills

- references—contact information for former employers who have been impressed with your work

If you don't put references on your résumé, have a separate list available for any interviewer who requests it.

In general, a good résumé is easy to read and neat (no coffee stains!), has no typos or spelling errors (proofread twice!), and explains to the potential employer why you are the person for the job without overstating your abilities.

COMPOSING THE COVER LETTER

You should always include a cover letter with every resume you send out. This will improve the odds that your resume will get the attention it deserves. A good cover letter is not, however, your résumé in paragraph form. Instead, use the cover letter to tell more about yourself, why you want that particular job, and why you would be good at it. Write a separate, individualized cover letter for each employer to whom you are sending your resume. Be sure to address it to the specific person or company to which you are applying.

ACING THE INTERVIEW

Think of your interview as your first day on the job. On your first day, you'll want to be on time, dressed appropriately, and ready to get started. For your interview, do what you need to do to appear ready to step into the position immediately.

Do:

- Be on time! Get the address and directions ahead of time, know where to park if you're driving, know how long it will take to get to the building at that time of day, and give yourself a little extra time to collect your thoughts as you walk to the office.

- Wear serious, modest clothing and look professional and competent.

- Bring a notebook and pen, in addition to extra copies of your résumé and list of references.

- Make pleasant eye contact, shake hands with confidence, and remember your interviewer's name.

- Ask questions. After all, you're trying to decide whether to work for them as much as they're trying to decide whether to hire you.

Did you notice that all of the items in this list sound familiar? That's because you've learned about all of these things in previous chapters on being a successful student. Now you're simply applying them in another setting!

Don't:

- Eat, drink, chew gum, wear headphones, or let your cell phone ring.

- Flirt or promise anything you can't deliver.

The bottom line is that your résumé, cover letter, and interview should be honest and confident. Don't oversell yourself, but don't sell yourself short either.

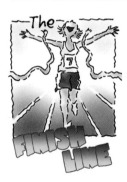

- Looking at how far you've come can be an encouragement to keep pursuing your dreams.

- It's important to celebrate every accomplishment, no matter how small.

- By thinking about the obstacles you've overcome so far, you can find ways to face future challenges.

- Evaluate how well you met your goals this semester or term and make plans to avoid problems in the future.

- The knowledge and skills you're learning now will be important to your future career in health care.

Review Questions

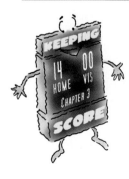

1. Short Essay: Write three to five sentences describing the dreams that brought you to where you are now.

2. What is the biggest obstacle you've overcome so far in your quest for a new career?

3. What goal are you most proud of accomplishing so far?

4. Short Essay: Write three to five sentences about the career knowledge you've gained since beginning school.

Chapter Activities

1. Assess Your Success: Make a timeline starting from when you first decided you wanted to pursue a health care career, and ending with your long-term goal. First, mark the steps you've taken so far, such as narrowing down your career choices, choosing a school, enrolling, registering for courses, adjusting your work schedule, etc. Then, add your intermediate and short term goals to the timeline. Finally, look at how far you've come and how much farther you need to go.

2. Share the Wealth: Divide into groups of three to five students. Ask each member of the group to talk about the fears he had when he first started school and how he found the courage to overcome those fears. Use a chalkboard or poster paper to make a list of fears and how each was overcome so everyone can take notes.

ANSWERS TO KEEPING SCORE QUESTIONS

CHAPTER 1   Review Questions

1. People may choose to continue their education to improve their lifestyles, provide for their families, and gain self-respect.

2. Answers will vary.

3. To be a successful student, look for support from friends and family, coworkers, other students, campus discussion groups, instructors and tutors, academic advisors, and campus resources.

4. Goals should be measurable, reachable, and desirable.

5. For questions about course requirements related to your degree or certificate plan, the best person to ask is an academic advisor.

Chapter Activities

1. Tasks may include but are not limited to:
   - Study the course catalog.
   - Meet with an academic advisor.
   - Register for classes.
   - Research information on financial aid.
   - Meet with a financial aid advisor.
   - Obtain a campus map.
   - Locate classrooms on campus.
   - Locate libraries, learning labs, and other campus resource centers.
   - Locate the campus bookstore and purchase books and supplies.

2. All areas located.

CHAPTER 2   Review Questions

1. You will get to know your instructors, take notes if your instructors lecture on the first day of class, find out about helpful campus resources, and receive important handouts.

2. Health professions classrooms tend to get noisy when instructors discuss clinical rotation assignments. If you are unable to hear your instructor over the conversations of other students, you won't know when or where to go for your clinical assignment.

3. They should be Committed Contributors who are Compatible with one another and Considerate of each other.

4. Learning how to meet and talk to new people now will help you feel more comfortable by the time you have your first real clinical experience.

5. Answers may include: Create a separate binder for each class to keep important paperwork in a safe place; keep your lecture notes for each class separate to avoid confusion; clean out your backpack every few days by filing stray papers in their appropriate binders.

Chapter Activities

1. Tasks could include:

   - Buy supplies (three-ring binders, tabbed dividers or colored card-stock paper, colored marker or pen, three-hole punch, spiral notebooks, etc.).
   - Designate a separate binder for each class.
   - Label tabbed dividers or card stock with appropriate headings (e.g., Schedule, Syllabus, Handouts, Assignments, Notes) and insert one set of dividers in each binder.
   - File all paperwork for each class behind the appropriate tabs.
   - Insert a supply of blank notebook paper behind the "Notes" tab in each binder (or use a separate spiral-bound notebook to take notes for each class).
   - Clean out your backpack after the first day of class. File any stray papers in their appropriate binders.

2. Each student has introduced someone.

CHAPTER 3   Review Questions

1. It gives you information about grading, homework assignments, course goals, and, sometimes, details about the course schedule.

2. Midterm and final exam dates; due dates for papers and other projects; deadlines for completing each phase of lengthy projects; test dates; your instructors' office hours; important extracurricular and recreational events; deadlines for drop/add; holidays, school vacations, and social commitments.

3. Answers will vary.

Chapter Activities

Answers will vary.

SPECIAL SECTION:

WHAT'S MY SCORE?   Grade Calculation Practice

1. 90.9%

2. 82.5%

3. 85%

4. 92.6%

5. 92%

CHAPTER 4   Review Questions

1. Answers may include: class discussions, class lectures, question-and-answer sessions, giving speeches, reading aloud, study groups, and recorded lectures or speeches.

2. Answers may include:

- Read aloud.

- Take notes or draw graphics as you read.

- Write down any questions you have about confusing concepts or ideas.

- Think about how information in the chapter relates to important points outlined in the table of contents (or outlined at the beginning of the chapter).

- Make a note of any difficult sections you'd like to read a second time.

3. Concept map.

4. Answers may include: summarize the information in your own words; begin memorizing key terms; predict which topics the instructor will cover next.

5. Assessment programs help students determine how much of the material they've learned. Students are then able to set goals that focus on their areas of weakness. These programs are helpful to instructors who can adjust their curricula according to the progress and needs of their students.

Chapter Activities

1. Answers will vary.
2. Answers will vary.

CHAPTER 5   Review Questions

1. Answers will vary but may include:
   - letting distractions interrupt your train of thought
   - tuning out difficult material
   - allowing your emotions to cloud your thinking
   - automatically assuming the material is boring
   - concentrating on the speaker's quirks
   - letting your mind wander
   - pretending to listen
   - only listening for facts and not ideas
   - trying to write down every word in your notes

2. Answers may include: interviews with professors or experts in the field, surveys and statistics, resources on the Internet, unbiased observations, personal experiences.

3. Answers will vary but should be similar to: Thinking critically means analyzing information in order to form judgments about it. The information may be gathered from observations, personal experience, reasoning, or communication.

Chapter Activities

1. Answers will vary.
2. Answers will vary.

CHAPTER 6   Review Questions

1. Answers will vary but may include: practice and repetition, spaced study, making associations, reducing interference, creating lists, or using imagery.

2. Answers will vary; sample answer: Possible challenges include finding trustworthy and helpful people to network with, getting up the nerve to approach them, and then finding a time when everyone is free to get together.

3. Answers will vary but may include: personal opinions, name-calling, outdated information, requests for the user's personal information.

Chapter Activities

1. Answers will vary but may include something similar to:

- a room where I can shut the door; a large desk so I can spread out my books and notes; a comfortable chair; a window; a CD player so I can listen to soft instrumental music
- move CD player from my bedroom to my study space; clear off the desk so I have room for my study materials; borrow some classical CDs from the local library

2. Answers will vary.

CHAPTER 7   Review Questions

1. Answers will vary but may include: Preparation is most important—study thoroughly, know what to study. Keep to your normal schedule, and don't cut out eating right or exercising. Budget your time well during the test and try to answer every question, even if only in outline form.

2. Talk to the instructor and look at old versions of the test.

3. When you're writing your outline, start with your thesis statement. Use the five-paragraph format to organize the body of your outline, including the introduction, your main points and supporting details, and your conclusion. It's important to write an outline because content and organization typically count for most of your test grade. If you run out of time and can't finish your essay, you can at least show your outline to let your instructor know that time was the problem, not comprehension.

Chapter Activities

1. List could include actions such as: I want to start riding my bike again and I want to try tai chi. For the bike, I'll need to get that front tire changed and buy a bike helmet. For tai chi, I could buy a video that shows me the basics, then practice it in the backyard.

2. Answers will vary.

CHAPTER 8   Review Questions

1. Use your school's skills lab.

2. If you try to do something you're not qualified to do, you could make a mistake and possibly harm a patient or get into legal trouble. But if you always work within your limits, you'll be protecting yourself, the patients, and the facility where you work.

3. Your mentor is someone who can be a role model, share her own experiences, answer your questions, and provide a private audience for your concerns.

Chapter Activities

1. Answers may vary but can include questions such as:
   - Where do I buy my uniform?
   - What happens if I accidentally break a HIPAA rule?
   - What if I make mistakes during a procedure?
2. Answers will vary.

CHAPTER 9   ### Review Questions

1. Answers will vary.
2. Answers will vary.
3. Answers will vary.
4. Answers will vary.

Chapter Activities

1. Answers will vary.
2. Answers will vary.

INDEX